Medical Disclaimer

Always consult your medical practitioner, registered dietician or nutritionist before making any significant changes to your diet – particularly if you are an adolescent, pregnant, breastfeeding or have or develop a medical condition.

Whilst our recipes can help most people lose weight as part of a calorie controlled diet and active lifestyle, they have not been specifically designed for you and individual results will vary.

Where calorie and macronutrient information is provided, it is calculated using common databases. Exact values will vary, however, and so the values will only be approximations for your finished dish.

Image credits (Hormone guide section):
Breakfast cereal: ifong©123RF.com; Snack bar: Baiba Opule©123RF.com; Sandwich: Sara Winter©123RF.com; Cookies: Mariusz Blach©123RF.com; Pasta Bake: Elena Veselova©123RF.com; Refined carbohydrates: akz©123RF.com; Sunshine: Nicola Zalewski©123RF.com; Sleeping Lady: Valeriy Lebedev©123RF.com; Chocolate Dessert: Elena Veselova©123RF.com

© Copyright 2021 The Health & Fitness Coach and its licensors

All rights reserved.
No part of this book may be reproduced, stored in a retrieval system or transmitted in any form or means whatsoever without the prior consent and written permission of the copyright holder(s).

CONTENTS

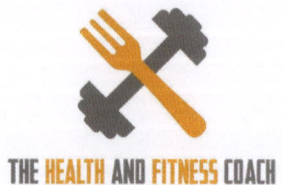

Introduction

Drinks

Banana choc chip smoothie	1
Coconut & lime frosty	2
Healthy veggie smoothie	3
Turkish delight inspired smoothie	4
Mint choc chip smoothie	5
Berry, banana & lime smoothie	6
Fruit & nut smoothie	7
Coconut dream smoothie	8

Snacks

Fruity frozen yoghurt	9
Sticky pear & chocolate squares	10
Nutty marmalade bars	11
Passion fruit cheesecake	12
Creamy coconut & cashew protein yoghurt	13
No bake brownies	14
Zesty chocolate fudge	15
Banana choc chip bars	16
Oaty cookies	17
Peanut & coconut energy balls	18
Beetroot, berry & chocolate cake	19
Peanut butter, chocolate & banana ice cream	20
Apple oaty bars	21
Coconut bliss energy balls	22

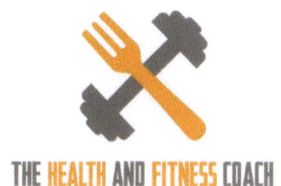

Breakfast

Berry banana smoothie bowl	23	Matcha smoothie bowl	35
Egg breakfast burrito	24	Chickpea breakfast hash	36
Oaty power bowl	25	Mexican scrambled eggs	37
Sweetcorn fritters topped with a poached egg	26	Mango overnight oats	38
		Strawberry cream porridge	39
Quick & easy protein pancakes	27	Egg breakfast bowl	40
Veggie-rich bake	28	Quick crunchy muesli	41
Breakfast bowl	29	Oatless nut porridge	42
Strawberry & almond overnight oats	30	Creamy baked eggs	43
		Feta & spinach breakfast hash	44
Baked oat cups	31	Fluffy berry omelette	45
Sweetcorn, spinach & chive muffins	32	Kale, bacon & egg fry up	46
		Scrambled eggs with a twist	47
Breakfast roasted peppers with eggs	33	Quinoa veggie bake	48
Mango & berry smoothie bowl	34		

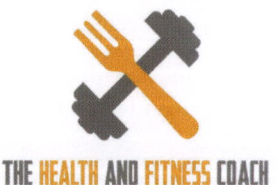

Lunch

Chicken fattoush	49	Cinammon chicken	62
Lemon & herb chicken	50	Sweet potato frittata	63
Courgetti carbonara	51	Lentil, cucumber & red pepper salad	64
Crustless tomato & basil quiche	52	Lemon cod fillets	65
Smokey chicken & mixed bean soup	53	Tuna stuffed courgette boats	66
		Chicken lentil soup	67
Blackened salmon with roasted vegetables	54	Dijon chicken wings	68
Carrot & coriander soup	55	Shish tawook	69
Vegan chickpea wraps	56	Chicken bulgur salad	70
Chipotle chicken & veggie bowl	57	Lentil kibbeh	71
BBQ chicken wings	58	Bulgur & butternut squash bowl	72
Salmon crustless quiche	59	Vegan scalloped potatoes	73
Egg salad	60	Caprese chicken salad	74
Red lentil soup	61		

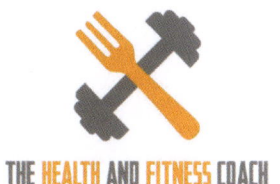

Dinner

Garlic & herb roast chicken	75	Veggie-rich ratatouille	89
Chicken in a creamy leek sauce	76	Baked chicken breast	90
		Fragrant chickpea burgers	91
Pan fried coconut & chilli fish with a spinach salad	77	Fragrant beef curry	92
Greek lamb chops	78	Quick Caribbean coconut prawns	93
Vegetarian moussaka	79	Hearty chicken casserole	94
Beef & lentil stew	80	Quick chicken & vegetable scramble	95
Chicken & vegetable pizza	81		
Roast cauliflower chicken	82	Stuffed cabbage	96
Mongolian beef	83	Easy cashew chicken	97
Stuffed aubergine	84	Herby baked salmon	98
Lamb curry	85	Spiced salmon & chickpea salad	99
Cauliflower burgers	86		
Chicken tagine with squash	87	Vegetable & chickpea paella	100
Chickpea curry	88		

Committed to your success
Rita, The Coach

WELCOME...

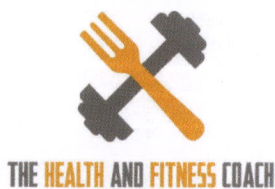

Welcome to **The Coach's Healthy Lifestyle Cookbook**.

This book will be your bible over the coming weeks! In case you didn't know, nutrition will count for about 80% of your results. That's right 80%! There is an important lesson to be learned from the story below...

You see I used to have a client, let's call her Lisa. Now Lisa trained very hard and never missed a training session and so with all this effort and dedication to her training she thought that the scales and the measuring tape would really be moving in the right direction at her weights and measurement day.

I will never forget the look on her face when she found out that she lost only ½kg and 2cms from her waist. She was disappointed and so was I.

"You have read the information on the importance of nutrition and you have been using the recipe book I gave you?" I asked. It turned out she never read it because she thought she already knew about nutrition and that her personal trainer wasn't going to know more than she did.

Sometimes we learn the hard way! I'm pleased to say that once Lisa had become fully aware of the importance of nutrition for fat loss, we were able to make some important changes. 28 days later she was 7kgs down and almost 2 dress sizes smaller.

As the saying goes, **"When the student is ready, the teacher will appear."**

And you are ready! That's why you are reading this!

The Coach xx

PRINCIPLES OF NUTRITION

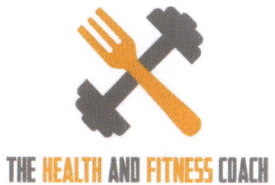

Below I have included the key principles that work for nutrition for health and fat loss. If anything you read, see or hear deviates from any of the six principles below, chances are you can dismiss it immediately as a short term fad diet. This is a way of eating that will enable you to achieve both fast and permanent results in a way that is 100% sustainable. You see this change has to be permanent so it has to be both straightforward and above all enjoyable. The good news is that my recipe book will show you how quick, easy and tasty eating this way is.

Follow these principles and you will get results...

1. Eating fewer calories than you burn (calorie deficit)
2. Eat more vegetables and fruits because they are rich in antioxidants and micro-nutrients (vitamins and minerals)
3. Eat plenty of protein for repair and maintenance of lean tissue, and to keep you feeling full (protein satisfies the appetite more than any other macronutrient)
4. Eat enough healthy fats from oily fish, nuts, avocados, coconut and olive oils (healthy fats are an essential part of a balanced diet)
5. Drink plenty of water to naturally detoxify the body, keeping the brain and body hydrated so it can function properly (green and herbal teas count towards this water intake)
6. Limit processed foods and artificial sweeteners and preservatives

Now go and learn, cook, and experience the benefits that my recipes have to offer – enjoy!

https://thehealthandfitnesscoach.co.uk

GET IN TOUCH

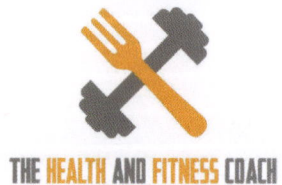

THE HEALTH AND FITNESS COACH

Website **https://thehealthandfitnesscoach.co.uk**

Email **rita@thehealthandfitnesscoach.co.uk**

Tel **+447769 690679**

- @RTHealthAndFitnessCoach
- the.health.and.fitness.coach
- @TheHealthandFi3

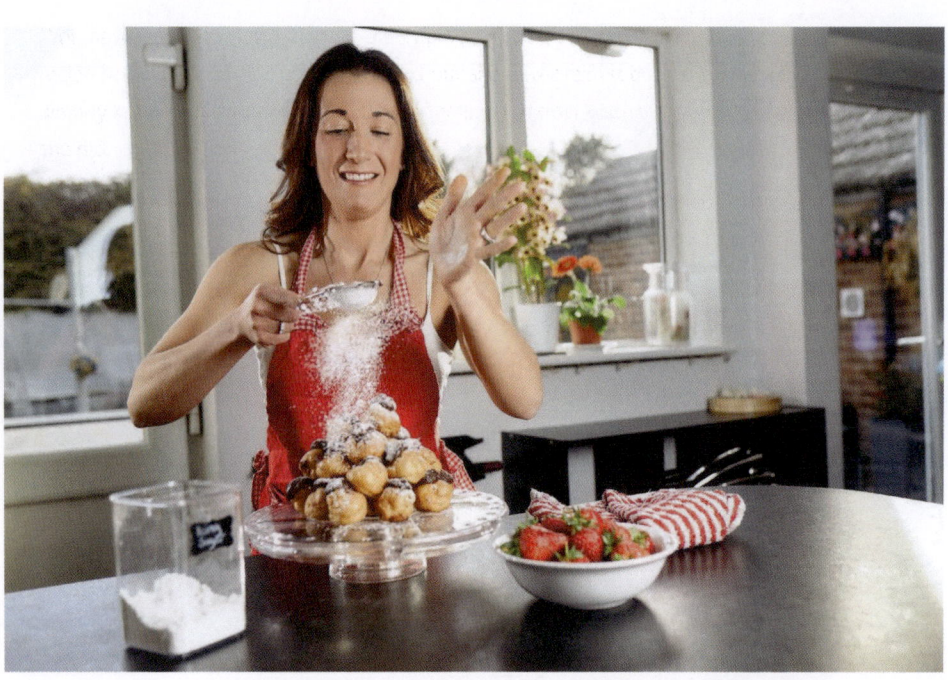

LET'S GET STARTED...

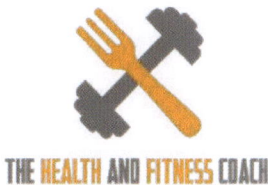

Below are a few hints and tips to help you along the way.
Please spare a few minutes to read this before you get cooking.

COOKING WITH FATS AND OILS

Coconut oil, olive oil and ghee are suitable for baking and shallow frying / sautéing. These fats are less likely to oxidise when cooking at medium / high temperatures.

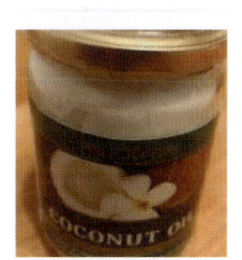

When oils oxidise, they become toxic, which can be damaging to your body.

Coconut oil is high in lauric acid, a fatty acid that is anti-fungal, anti-bacterial and anti-viral.

If you are following a dairy free diet, it is best to cook with coconut oil or olive oil.

When ghee is made, the milk solids are almost completely removed, therefore ghee is often suitable for people who are lactose intolerant.

For salads, use cold pressed extra virgin olive oils, sesame or peanut oils.

There are also a variety of fats and oils that should be avoided completely. All hydrogenated and partially hydrogenated oils are bad for you and can contribute to a range of serious health problems such as cancer, heart disease and immune dysfunction.

COCONUT FLOUR

A gluten free alternative to normal flour. This is a versatile ingredient, which can be used in baking and cooking. Makes great pancakes!

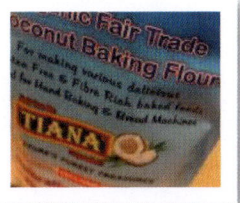

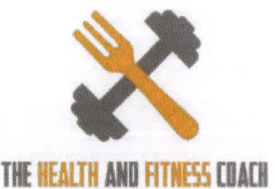

TEA

Green tea has lots of amazing health benefits. It is high in antioxidants and contains about half the amount of caffeine of normal tea. It is widely available in supermarkets, health shops and online.

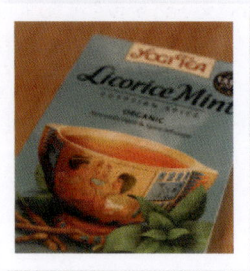

Tulsi Brahmi (caffeine free) is another healthy alternative with healing properties, as well as also being a rich source of antioxidants.

Of all herbal teas, liquorice tea is arguably one of the most beneficial yet under-appreciated herbal teas. Liquorice tea can help the liver to rid the body of unwanted toxins, can relieve constipation, is used to treat low blood pressure, helps to lower cholesterol and is an anti-allergenic so is helpful for hay fever and conjunctivitis sufferers.

STORECUPBOARD SAVIOURS

There are plenty of simple ways to make your food taste good. Why not keep your cupboards stocked up with a handy supply of spices and rubs, which are generally very cheap to buy, simple to use, and a much healthier alternative to the artificial flavourings, additives and sugars found in many of the processed sauces available.

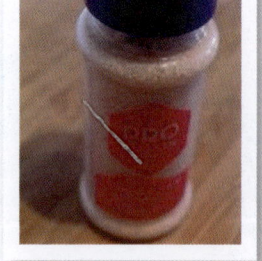

Consider replacing cheap, processed table salt (which is full of chemicals and some even contain sugar!) with a good quality organic sea salt or Himalayan pink salt. This salt contains many beneficial minerals and can help balance electrolytes, eliminate toxins and support nutrient absorption.

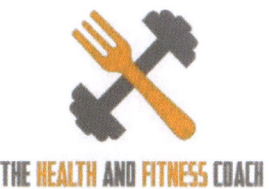

A LITTLE SWEETNESS

Sugar gets a lot of bad press these days due to the negative effects it can have on your health. For example, excessive consumption suppresses the immune system and reduces insulin sensitivity.

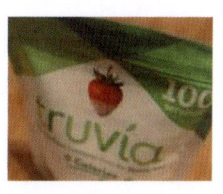

However, I believe it is important to consider the for and against, and not just react to what we see in the news. If you lead a healthy lifestyle, eat a balanced, varied diet, and enjoy moderate regular exercise, then there really shouldn't be cause for panic.

Within the huge category that sugar spans, are a range of good and bad food choices. If, for example, you cut out all fruit for the rest of your life (because fruit contains sugar), you might well miss out on some key nutrients. Plus you may feel deprived.

My advice to you is that it is your choice if you consume sugar and/or sugar alternatives. But what is probably more important is to consider that worrying about the matter could be equally bad or even worse for your health. Instead, why not try to look at sugar and sugar alternatives as a 'treat' rather than a necessity... something to really savour and enjoy every once in a while (without the guilt!).

In some of my recipes, I have used natural sweeteners such as Stevia. Many research studies have been conducted on the safety of these products and while no definite links have been made to any negative health effects, overall the evidence for and against it is still inconclusive. If you'd prefer to swap the sweeteners in these recipes with something else then feel free to do so. Home made apple sauce, raisins and bananas can add enough sweetness to a variety of baking recipes.

Note: There are several forms of Stevia available - a very light powdery texture, and a more granulated/grainy texture. In all of my recipes, I have used the granulated version. I recommend you use the same, so that the ingredient weight is accurate.

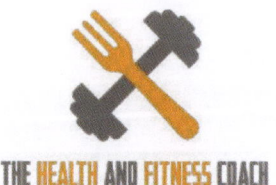

FLAXSEED

Flaxseed is rich in omega-3 fatty acids and fibre. It is a great ingredient to use in cooking and baking, e.g. spelt bread, cakes, pizzas (yes, healthy ones!), mixed in with nut butter or humous dips, added to pancake mixes, sprinkled over cereals or salads or added to smoothies.

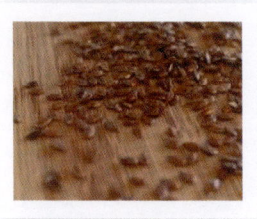

It's best to grind the flaxseed up in a coffee grinder first, as it is not absorbed by the body if left whole. If you mix flaxseed with water and leave to stand for 10 minutes, it develops a sticky coating, which makes it a great egg substitute in baking (as do chia seeds). Always store your flaxseed in the fridge in an airtight container.

WHITE OR WHOLEGRAIN RICE?

Generally speaking, wholegrain, unprocessed carbohydrates tend to be better handled than processed carbohydrates such as white rice, pasta, bread and cereals.

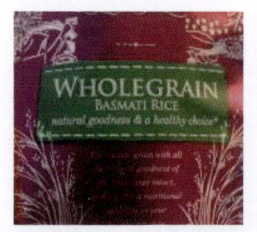

Wholegrain rice is probably a healthier option than white rice, nevertheless it should still be consumed in moderation, especially if you are trying to lose fat. In most cases, where rice appears in this book, I haven't specified white or wholegrain rice. Please decide for yourself which is the best option for you.

A HELPING HAND...

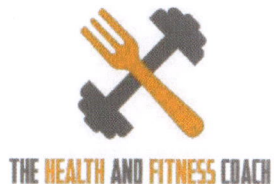

Through a combination of good nutrition and exercise, the following recipes will help you achieve optimum fat loss results.

Here are some low carb recipes, ideal for a **non training day:**

Breakfast
- Quick & easy protein pancakes
- Veggie-rich bake
- Sweetcorn, spinach & chive muffins
- Mexican scrambled eggs

Lunch & Dinner
- Chicken fattoush
- Lemon & herb chicken
- Crustless tomato & basil quiche
- Blackened salmon with roasted vegetables
- Salmon crustless quiche
- Egg salad
- Shish tawook
- Garlic & herb roast chicken
- Greek lamb chops

Snacks & Treats
- Peanut & coconut energy balls
- Buckwheat, cranberry & pistachio bites
- Creamy coconut & cashew protein yoghurt
- Zesty chocolate fudge

Smoothies
- Cardamom & mint lassi
- Mint choc chip smoothie

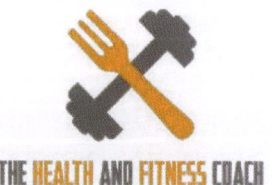

Research has shown that the body can tolerate carbohydrate better after exercise. If you are going to consume carbs, you should aim to do this within 2 hours of exercise.

Here are some recipes which are ideal post-workout. Many of these are also medium / high protein to aid muscle repair.

Breakfast
- Berry banana smoothie bowl
- Oaty power bowl
- Strawberry & almond overnight oats
- Chickpea breakfast hash

Lunch & Dinner
- Smokey chicken & mixed bean soup
- BBQ chicken wings
- Vegan chickpea wraps
- Chipotle chicken & veggie bowl
- Lentil kibbeh
- Chicken tagine with squash
- Hearty chicken casserole
- Quick chicken & vegetable scramble

Snacks & Treats
- Sticky pear & chocolate squares
- No bake brownies
- Banana choc chip bars
- Oaty cookies

Smoothies
- Berry, banana & lime smoothie
- Fruit & nut smoothie

GUIDE TO HORMONES

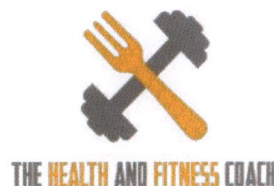

Understanding how hormones work and how our lifestyle choices affect our hormone levels, is vital if we want to get the best results possible. In fact I'd go as far to say that if our hormones are not regulated properly, it can massively sabotage our results and lead to poor health.

Obesity, diabetes and depression are just a few of the diseases that hormonal imbalances contribute towards. Whilst the diagnosis and treatment of hormonal imbalances should be left to medical experts, we can have a positive impact on our hormones by leading a healthy lifestyle.

A basic understanding of the key hormones that regulate metabolism, hunger, body fat, and energy levels is useful for understanding how different lifestyle choices affect your body.

Every time we eat, exercise, sleep, get stressed or meditate; hormones are released.

We want to make sure that our lifestyle choices help us to optimise the way our hormones are working.

What are hormones?

Hormones are chemical messengers that communicate information throughout the body.

You could think of hormones as radio signals that tell different cells in the body to do different things.

Depending on our lifestyle choices, the hormones released will dictate whether we burn or store body fat, feel hungry or satisfied, build muscle or not, feel relaxed or stressed, and whether we are able to sleep well or have restless nights.

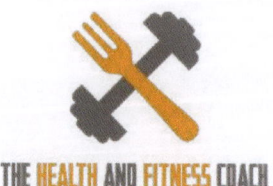

Can you see why this is so important to your health and the results you want to achieve? On the next few pages, we are going to look at a variety of different hormones that influence our health and our body composition. Let's get started...

Insulin

Insulin is released from the pancreas in response to raised blood glucose and increased energy intake. Skimmed milk is more insulinemic than white bread, so insulin is not just a blood glucose hormone. When our blood sugars increase, insulin is released and its job is to tell the body to store the sugar in our muscles and liver. Insulin transiently inhibits the release of lipids from fat tissue, but even with multiple insulin spikes, energy balance is the sole dictator of fat loss.

To slow the rate in which food leaves the stomach, the majority of our carbohydrate sources should be coming from fibre-rich whole grains. Added sugars offer no nutritional benefits, and so should be minimised but not demonised, as this can lead to poor relationships around food. Insulin's role is to prevent glucose remaining in the blood, as this is toxic. Its role is to move the glucose away from the blood.

The "blood sugar rollercoaster" and the often talked about "crash" is known as *reactive hypoglycemia* and is very rare in non-diabetics. Insulin is actually an anorexogenic hormone, which means it fills you up. Higher insulin releases after meals are associated with increased satiety. This "crash" is often due to postprandial somnolence, which is simply the digestive energy requirement of digesting a large meal. The craving for more sugary food is most likely not due to the drop in blood sugar, but the body craving more easily obtained energy in the form of sugar.

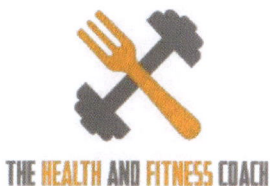

How popular food choices affect energy levels and hunger:

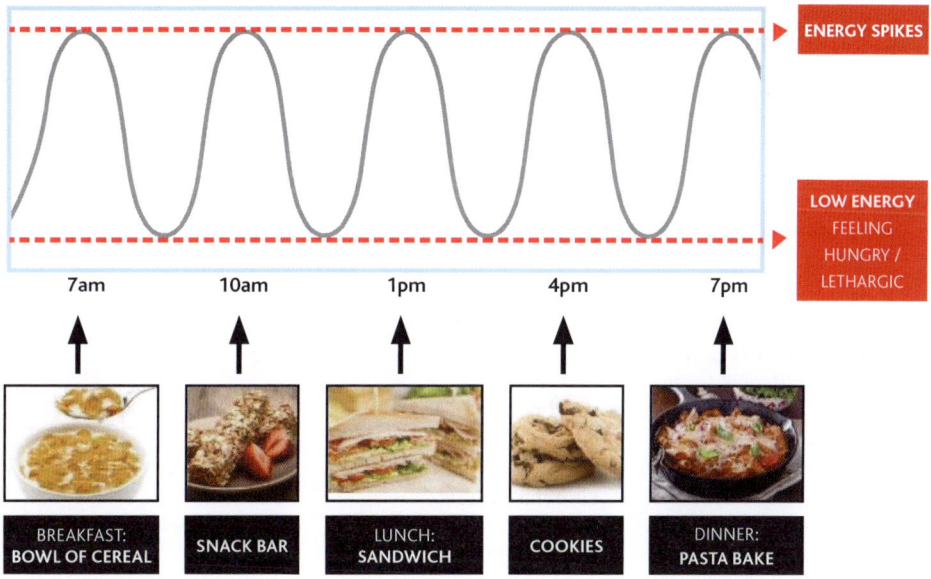

From a fat loss perspective, energy balance should be the key focus. However maintaining good blood glucose control can reduce our risk of metabolic syndrome and diabetes. How well we regulate blood glucose is due to carbohydrate type, fitness level, muscle mass and genetics.

Protein can actually have a higher insulin response than white bread. Both whey protein and skimmed milk stimulate larger releases of insulin. Fibre will slow the rate of gastric emptying and reduce the glycemic load of a meal, while fats on their own, do not raise blood glucose. A combination of carbohydrate and fat will slow down gastric emptying.

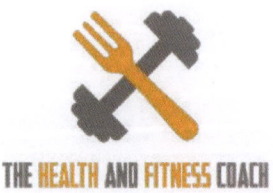

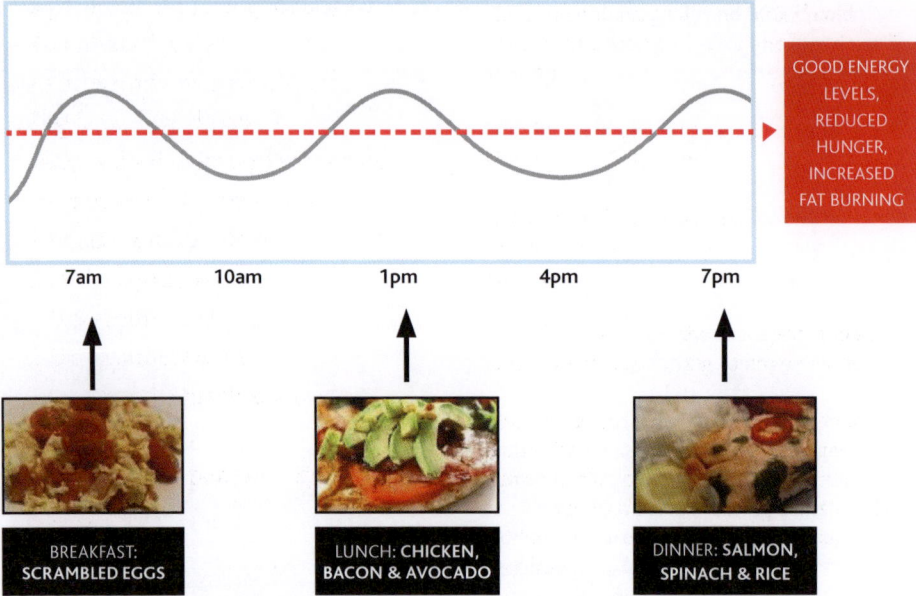

Insulin resistance is characterised by either the pancreas secreting too much insulin, or skeletal muscle failing to respond the the effects of insulin. It is a myth that eating too much sugar causes insulin resistance. A cell becoming resistant to insulin is multifaceted and the main culprit is prolonged energy excess in combination with inactivity.

An inactive muscle is less sensitive to the effects of insulin. This can lead to increased likelihood of a build up of serum blood glucose, as the muscle cannot properly utilise the glucose. We then need our pancreas to produce more insulin to shift the same amount of sugar out of the blood and into storage. This can be the beginning of metabolic syndrome and Type 2 diabetes.

The two main culprits behind insulin resistance are a lack of exercise and a hyper-caloric diet high in refined carbohydrates. The good news is that insulin sensitivity can be regained with the right combination of diet and exercise.

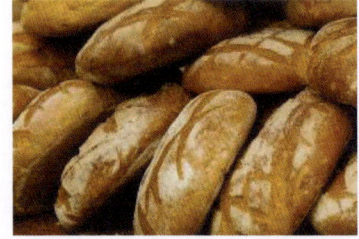

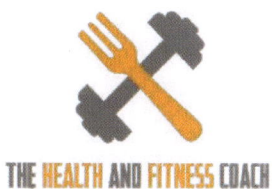

Glucagon

If we think of insulin as a **"storage hormone,"** then we can think of glucagon as a **"mobilisation hormone."**

Glucagon tells our muscle and fat cells to release energy for us to use to fuel our daily activities. If we consume a surplus of Calories and lots of sugary carbohydrates, glucagon doesn't need to do its job, because there's already too much energy available. Insulin and glucagon are both released from the pancreas and work with each other to regulate our blood sugars and energy levels. If our insulin levels are chronically high, this could increase our risk of Type 2 diabetes and metabolic syndrome. When our insulin levels are low, this signals to the body that energy availability is low. If we have poor blood glucose control, this may lead to increased appetite and a sudden urge to eat, which is the reactive hypoglycemia mentioned earlier.

In a nutshell, by eating the right foods to prevent insulin spikes, glucagon can do what we want it to do; help us to use our fat stores for energy.

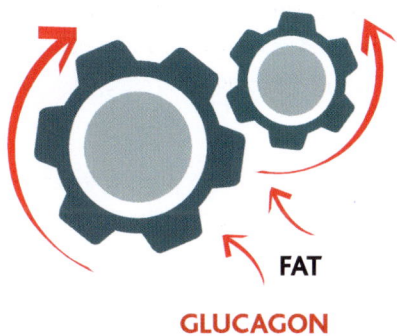

GLUCAGON

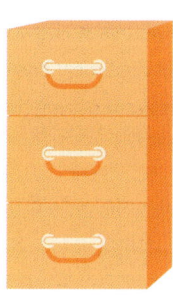

INSULIN

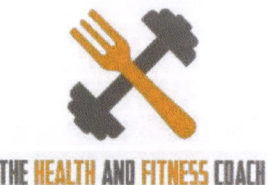

Cortisol

Cortisol is a hormone that is released from the adrenal glands (along with adrenaline). Although cortisol gets a bad wrap, it's actually very necessary for us to have cortisol, just not chronically elevated levels or unhealthy cortisol rhythms.

It's usually described as a stress hormone because we release cortisol (and adrenaline) in stressful situations. If we didn't release cortisol in the morning, then we would struggle to wake up.

Adrenaline tends to be an instant reaction, whereas cortisol works more slowly. Cortisol is a glucocorticoid hormone, so its job is to increase blood glucose to ensure we have an available supply during periods of stress.

Cortisol levels should rise in the mornings so that we feel energetic in the daytime, and gradually lower throughout the day, enabling us to feel relaxed and naturally tired in the evenings.

Modern life can be stressful and if, for example, we are stressing out over a work situation at night, then our cortisol levels can become elevated at a time when they should be low. Overtraining can also cause our cortisol levels to become chronically elevated so it's important that our training programmes are assessed regularly.

How healthy cortisol levels look:

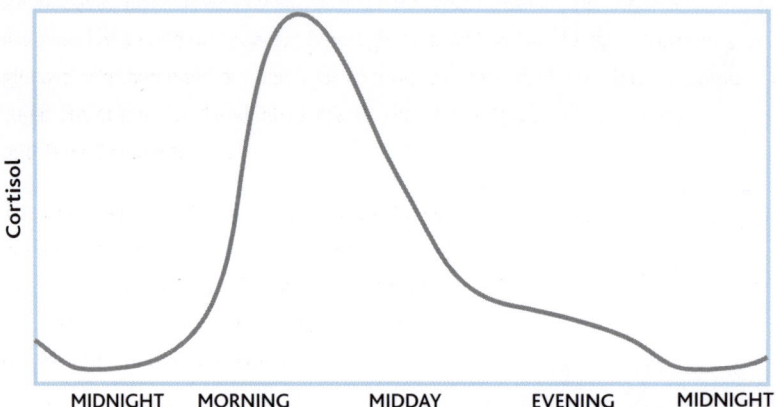

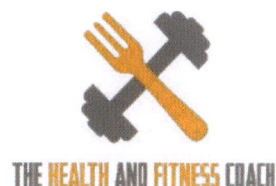

Some of the reasons that our cortisol levels become imbalanced:

- Poor sleeping habits
- Inability to handle or manage stress
- Overconsumption of stimulants; caffeine for example
- Overtraining; training too long / frequently at high intensity

When cortisol gets out of control, we can experience suppressed immune system function, elevated blood sugars, faster ageing and poor insulin sensitivity. This is the perfect recipe for getting sick, overweight and wrinkly. Times of stress often see us reaching for convenient sugary foods that taste good. Stress can often lead to comfort eating, but everyone deals with stress in different ways, so cortisol does not directly cause weight gain, but behaviours associated with stress could.

Things that can help to restore healthy cortisol levels:

- Getting 6-9 hours of good quality sleep every night
- Learning a cognitive strategy such as CBT to learn how to cope better with stress
- Taking time to meditate / relax / chill out more often
- Reducing caffeine intake, especially in the afternoons
- Ensuring your training regimen is assessed regularly

Growth hormone

Human growth hormone has been described as **"the fountain of youth"** and not surprisingly growth hormone supplementation is now big business, especially in the USA. **Good growth hormone levels help to keep us lean, healthy and strong.** As we age, our levels of growth hormone decline. For example, a 60 year old may only produce 25% of the growth hormone of a 20 year old. In that sense, there's not a lot we can do, because we're all getting older. What we can do, however, is to look at ways to help our bodies produce growth hormone normally and naturally.

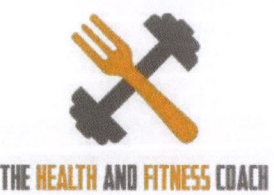

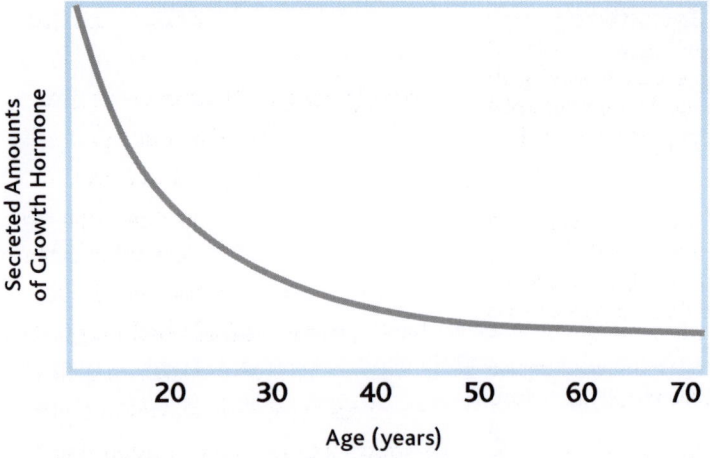

Growth hormone is mainly released / elevated when we are:

- Sleeping
- Exercising
- Fasting

If we are not sleeping properly, not only is our cortisol rhythm disturbed, we also miss out on our natural growth hormone release during sleep. This is another great reason to get to bed early and to watch our caffeine intake.

Exercise causes the release of growth hormones, so if we are exercising regularly then our bodies will be producing growth hormones naturally. Fasting also increases growth hormone levels, which is one of the reasons intermittent fasting has become popular. Whether or not you should fast is an individual decision and it's important to note that although it can increase growth hormone, it can also increase cortisol levels, so if you're already stressed, then fasting might not be the best option.

In terms of muscle gain, fasting is not an anabolic process. Fasting will initiate certain processes in the body like AMPK and autophagy, which are both catabolic clearance of damaged cells and mitochondria. Eating too many sugary carbohydrates can also lower growth hormone, yet another reason to ditch the junk foods.

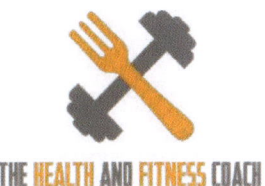

Testosterone

Although testosterone is the dominant male sex hormone, it is produced by both men and women. **Healthy testosterone levels are associated with drive, motivation and virility.** As we age, testosterone production declines and this contributes to the loss of muscle mass that people experience as they age. Low testosterone levels are associated with increased risk of cardiovascular diseases, depression, lethargy and lack of motivation.

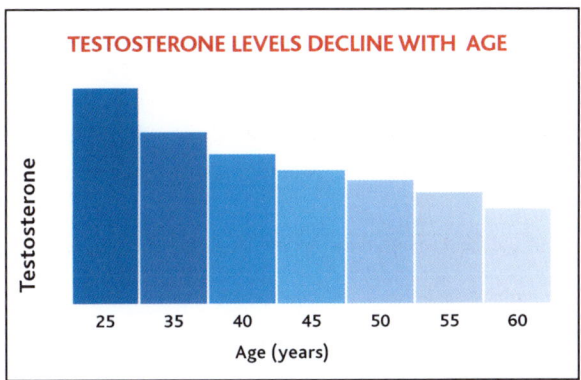

It is to be expected that certain hormones decline with age, in fact it's completely normal and natural, but what is a concern is the generational decline in testosterone levels in males. Our grandfathers, on average would have had much higher testosterone levels throughout their lives.

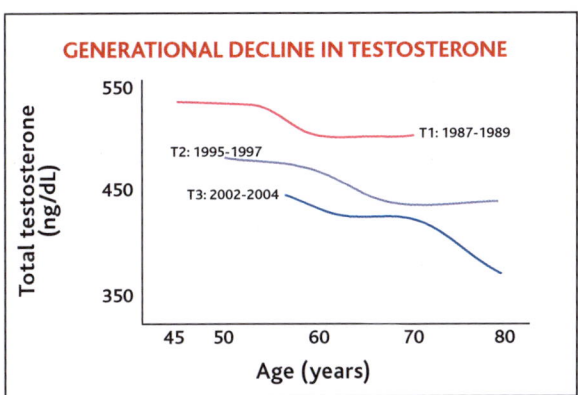

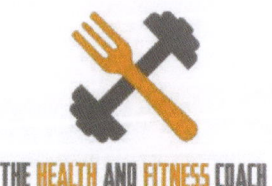

One of the reasons for this is that modern life can be a lot more stressful. So it's not that surprising when we see studies showing that cortisol blocks the effects of testosterone.

What can we do?

Luckily there are things we can do to maintain healthy testosterone levels:

- Get to bed early
- Learn stress management techniques
- Train with heavy weights
- Eat enough fat (our bodies make testosterone from cholesterol)

Training with heavy weights will not cause women to look big and bulky because females have a very small amount of testosterone compared to males, as the table below shows.

TOTAL TESTOSTERONE LEVELS		
SEX	ng/dl	ng/ml
Females	6-86	0.1-1.2
Males	270-1100	1.4-12

This explains the difference in ability between men and women to build muscle mass. It also explains why some men find it easier than other men to build muscle. The normal range has a huge variance, so a man sitting naturally at 1000+ will find it easier to build muscle than a man with low 200s.

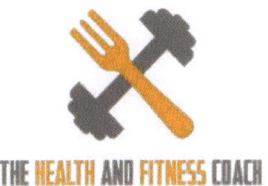

Oestrogen

It's often thought that information about oestrogen is only relevant to females. Oestrogen however, is an important topic for any man experiencing the dreaded "man boobs" or "moobs". **Men need a normal, healthy level of oestrogen just as women need a normal healthy level of testosterone.** The problem arises when oestrogen becomes out of balance with testosterone. This is when men can literally start growing what look like breasts. Obesity, as well as exposure to environmental oestrogens such as plastics, are thought to contribute towards the disruption of healthy sex hormone levels in males.

For women, healthy oestrogen levels are essential for heart and bone health, as well as many other functions in the body.

Estradiol is the primary oestrogen that a woman relies upon during her younger years to keep her healthy and lean. Estradiol also helps to regulate appetite, mood and energy levels. As a woman goes through the menopause, production of estradiol decreases and this leaves another form of oestrogen, estrone, as the main oestrogen. Estrone is linked with increased abdominal fat storage and unfortunately, the more fat that is gained, the more estrone is produced. This can make losing body fat much more difficult, and extra attention must be placed upon diet and exercise during and after the menopause. Estrone can also contribute to insulin resistance, another good reason to avoid bingeing on sugary carbohydrates and opt instead for proteins, fats, vegetables and complex carbohydrates.

Estradiol is also vital for calcium synthesis, and this is why women who have been through the menopause will require more calcium.

Another hormone that drops at the menopause is **progesterone**. Because progesterone is a precursor for testosterone and estradiol, this now means that there is less testosterone and estradiol available to have a positive effect on body composition, mood and appetite regulation. This is why it's so important to do everything within our control to promote healthy body composition, mood and appetite regulation. We can do this by paying attention to diet, exercise and stress levels.

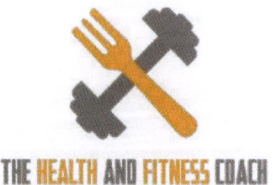

Chronically elevated cortisol levels around the time of the menopause need to be avoided, because cortisol and progesterone may compete for the same receptors. This means that cortisol can exhibit a blocking affect on progesterone. This is definitely not good if we consider progesterone levels are already dramatically lowered after the menopause.
The key message is to learn how to manage stress and make the right lifestyle choices.

Thyroid

Thyroid hormone is often referred to as "the master hormone" and with good reason. Thyroid hormones have a huge impact on metabolic rate. If you or anyone you know has suffered with under-active thyroid, then you know all about the weight gain and lethargy that can be experienced when the thyroid isn't functioning optimally. On the contrary, when the thyroid is over-active, people lose weight rapidly and can become anxious.
Important nutrients for thyroid health include; iodine, selenium, vitamin D3 and vitamin B12.

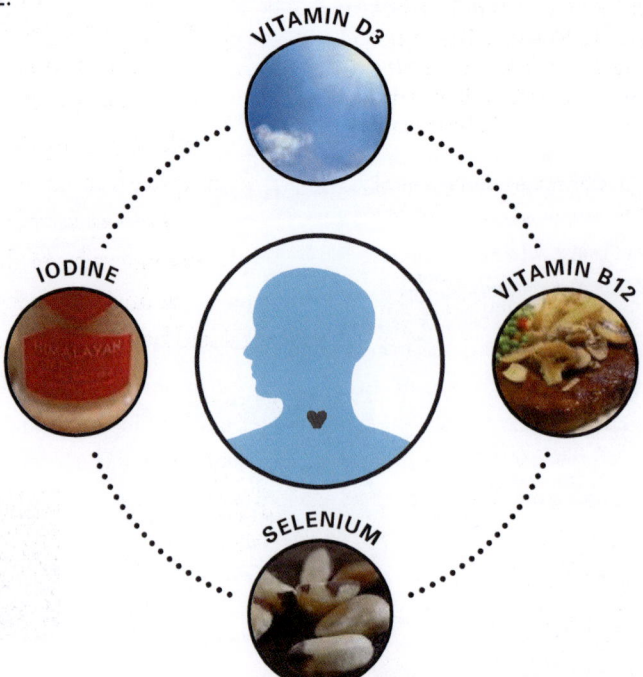

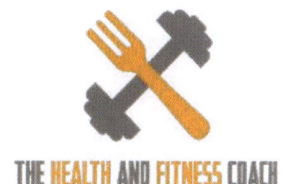

Cruciferous vegetables such as broccoli contain substances called goitrogens that inhibit the thyroid gland. Most of these substances are destroyed by cooking, so it's important to cook your cruciferous vegetables.

Leptin

Leptin is a hormone that decreases hunger by signalling to the brain that we have enough energy (fat) stores in our body. The problem is that, as in the case with insulin resistance, we can become resistant to leptin. The leaner someone is, the more sensitive to leptin they are, so a small amount of leptin does the job of telling us we're not hungry. This makes sense when we consider that leaner people actually have less leptin, even though they have less energy (fat) stored in their bodies.

When someone is leptin resistant, although they may have more leptin, the message doesn't get through and the result is feeling hungry. Not sleeping properly can also decrease leptin levels.

What can we do?

- Take Omega 3 fish oil – Omega 3 fats are associated with decreased hunger
- Go to bed early
- Reduce stress
- Reduce caffeine

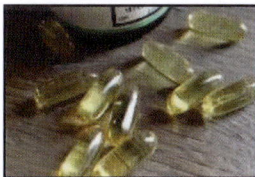 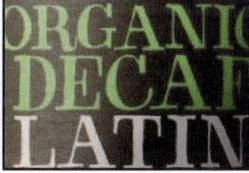 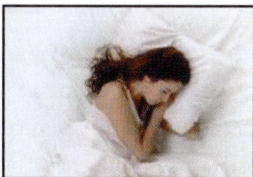

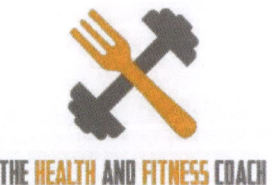

Ghrelin

Ghrelin is the hormone that tells us we are hungry. When it's coming up to meal time, we will naturally feel hungry, because ghrelin is being released. There's not a whole lot we can do to directly influence ghrelin, apart from, you guessed it, sleep well! Studies show that just 2 hours less sleep can increase ghrelin by 27%.

It's not only leptin and ghrelin that regulate our appetite, so we still can put practices into place to help us get our appetite under control.

There are other ways to help:

- Consume fibre-rich foods to help keep us feeling full
- Consume enough protein and fat because these two nutrients help to satiate us more than carbohydrates
- Drink enough water – sometimes when we think we are hungry, we're really just thirsty
- Free sugar containing foods are often not as satiating, so it is likely beneficial to mimimise consumption.

 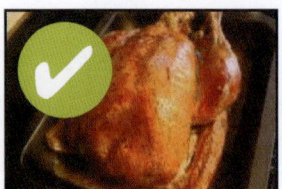 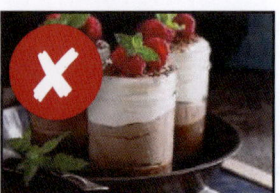

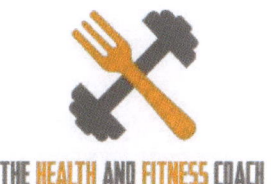

Conclusion

There are many hormones in the body, all having unique actions in maintaining sound health. The interplay between all the different hormones is complex, and while we don't need to understand everything about hormones, we can conclude that **the right lifestyle choices play a huge role in balancing our hormones.**

To help balance all of our hormones naturally we need to:

- Ensure that we are getting adequate amounts of good quality sleep
- Learn strategies to cope better with stress
- Taking time to meditate / relax / chill out
- Ensure we are not constantly overtraining
- Perform resistance training
- Reduce caffeine intake

Please be aware that this information does not constitute medical advice. If you are concerned about your hormonal health, please see a qualified medical professional.

Banana choc chip smoothie

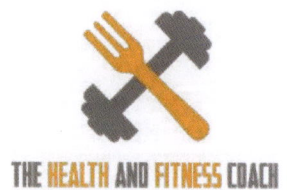

170ml unsweetened almond milk (or use milk of your choice)
70g frozen banana
30g vanilla or banana flavour whey or rice protein powder
40g Greek yoghurt (use dairy free if preferred)
2 tsps cocoa nibs
4 ice cubes

SERVES 1

Place all of the ingredients in a blender and blend until smooth. Serve.

Consume immediately.

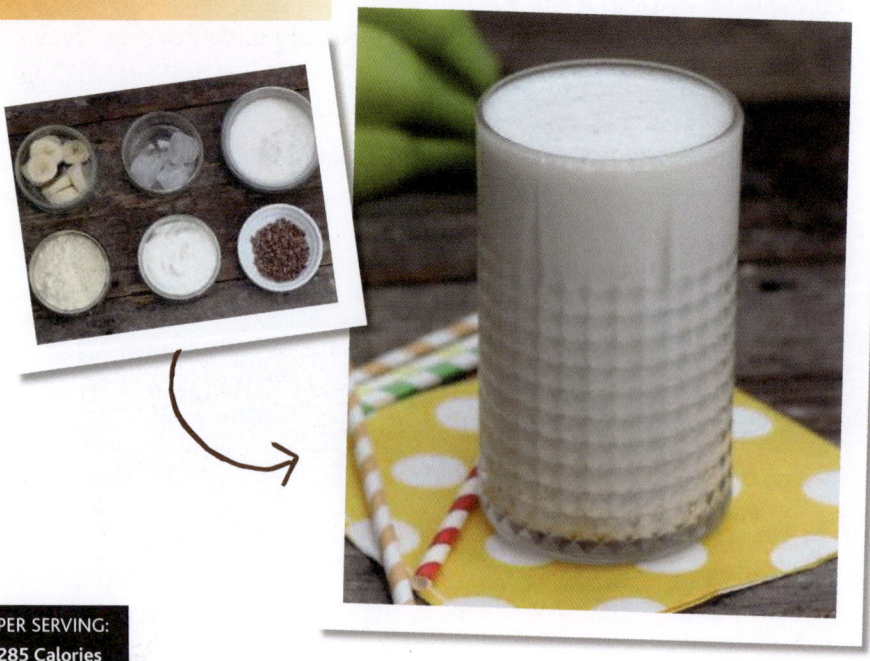

PER SERVING:
285 Calories
21g Carbs
30g Protein
9g Fat

https://thehealthandfitnesscoach.co.uk   DRINKS

Coconut & lime frosty

50g frozen banana
120ml long life coconut drink or unsweetened almond milk
50ml coconut milk (chilled or frozen)
juice of ½ a lime (optional)
1 tsp vanilla extract or vanilla bean paste
25g vanilla or coconut flavour whey or rice protein powder
1 tsp desiccated coconut
8-10 ice cubes

SERVES 1

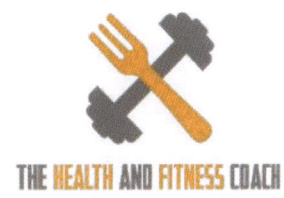

Place all of the ingredients in a blender and blend until creamy. Serve.

Consume immediately.

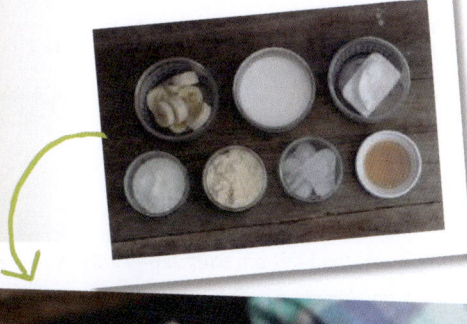

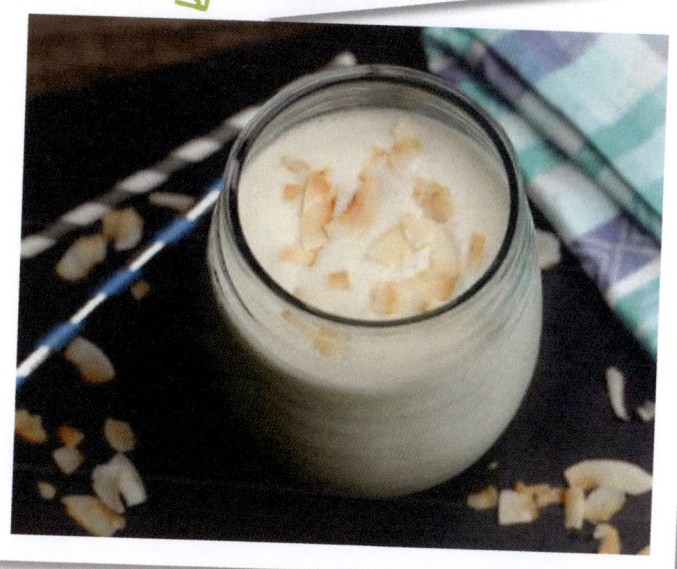

PER SERVING:
263 Calories
21g Carbs
20g Protein
11g Fat

https://thehealthandfitnesscoach.co.uk — DRINKS

Healthy veggie smoothie

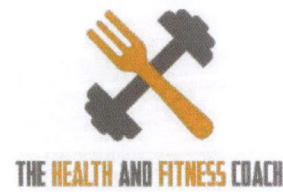

THE HEALTH AND FITNESS COACH

220ml unsweetened almond milk
60g frozen banana
1 medium-sized carrot, peeled
30g vanilla flavour whey or rice protein powder
1 tsp fresh ginger
¼ tsp ground turmeric
½ tsp ground cinnamon
¼ tsp ground black pepper (optional)
1 tsp chia seeds

SERVES 1

Place all of the ingredients in a blender and blend until smooth. Serve.

Consume immediately.

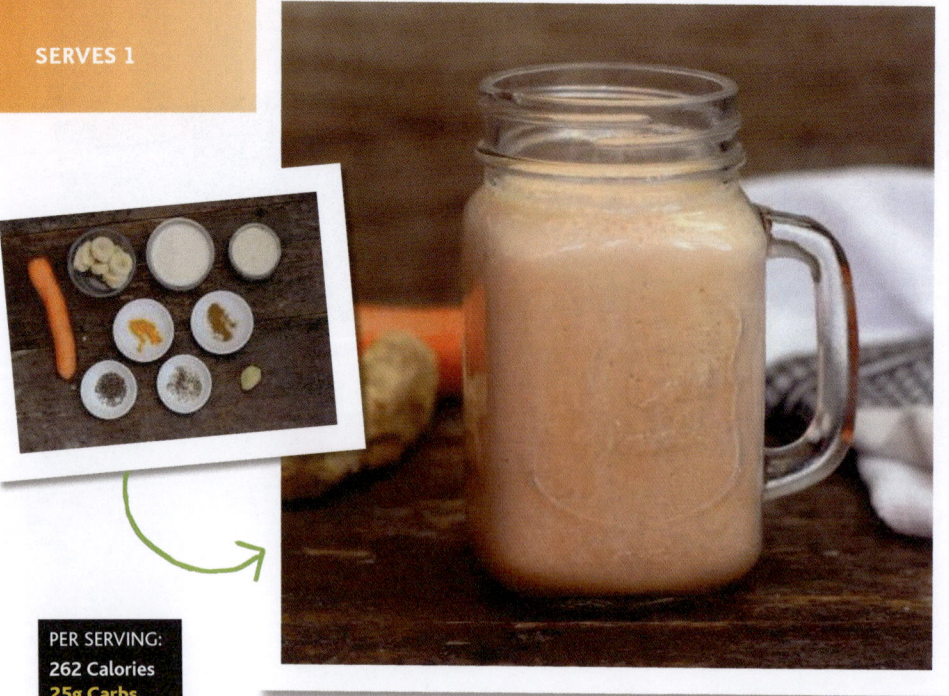

PER SERVING:
262 Calories
25g Carbs
27g Protein
6g Fat

https://thehealthandfitnesscoach.co.uk

Turkish delight inspired smoothie

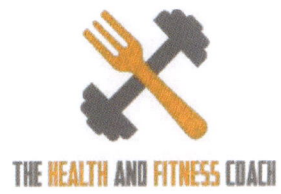

250ml unsweetened almond milk
40g frozen avocado
60g Greek yoghurt (use dairy free if preferred)
40g frozen banana
25g vanilla flavour whey or rice protein powder
5g shelled pistachios
2 tsps rose water

SERVES 1

Place all of the ingredients in a blender and blend until creamy. Serve.

Consume immediately.

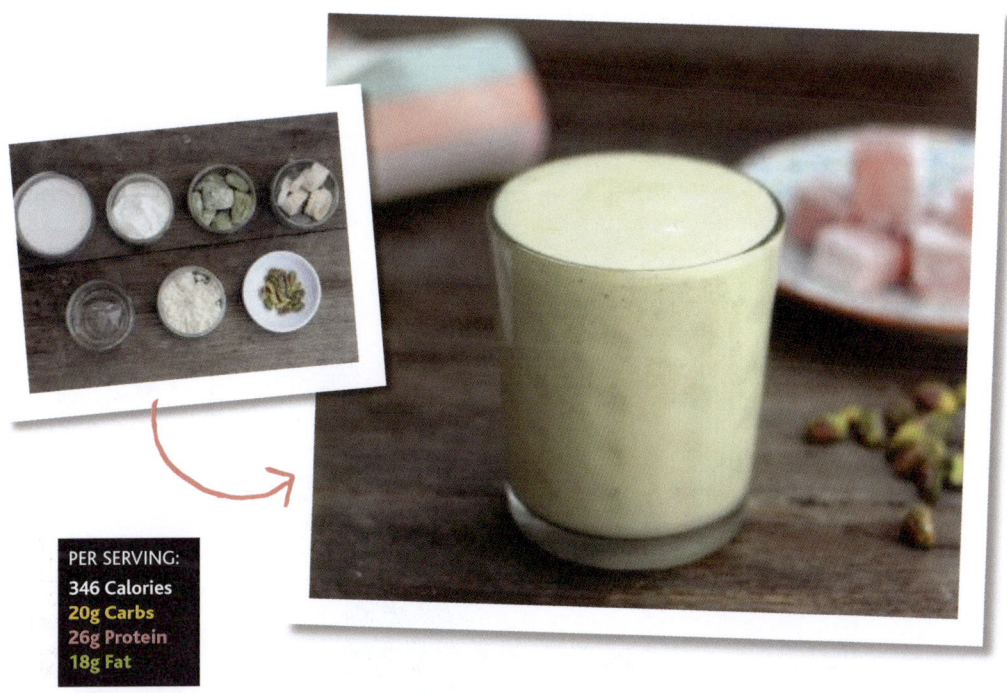

PER SERVING:
346 Calories
20g Carbs
26g Protein
18g Fat

https://thehealthandfitnesscoach.co.uk

Mint choc chip smoothie

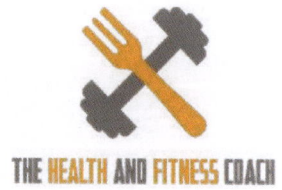

for the mint layer:
30g frozen avocado
a large handful of spinach leaves
½ tsp mint extract
15g vanilla flavour whey or rice protein powder
120ml unsweetened almond milk
1 tsp cocoa nibs

for the chocolate layer:
40g frozen banana
15g chocolate flavour whey or rice protein powder
2 tbsps cocoa powder
120ml unsweetened almond milk

SERVES 1

Place the mint layer ingredients into a blender jug and blend well until smooth. Pour into a glass.

Rinse the blender jug. Place the chocolate layer ingredients into the jug and blend well until smooth.

Pour the chocolate layer over the mint layer. Serve.

Consume immediately.

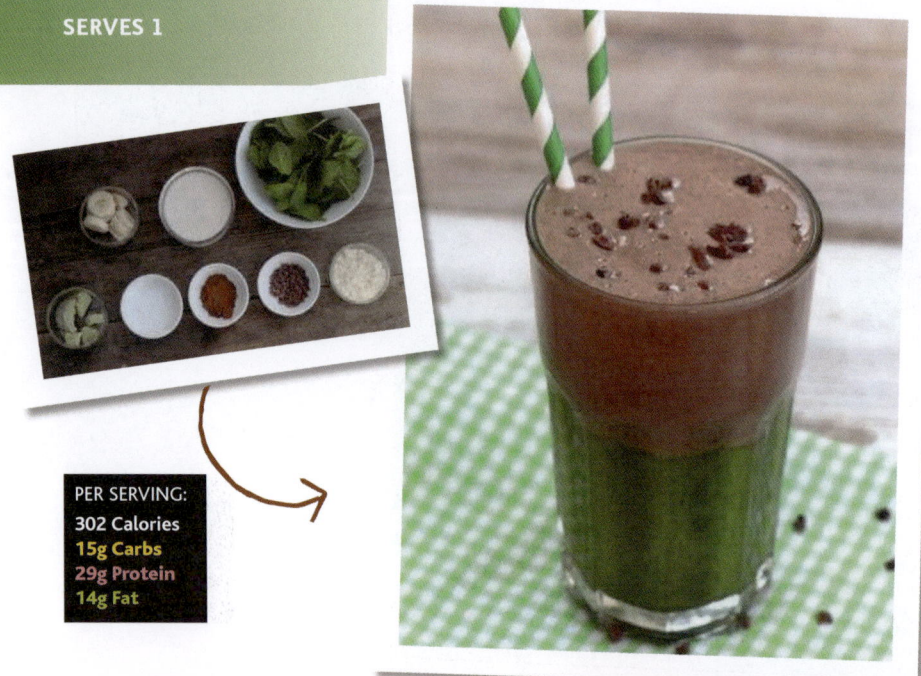

PER SERVING:
302 Calories
15g Carbs
29g Protein
14g Fat

https://thehealthandfitnesscoach.co.uk   DRINKS   5

Berry, banana & lime smoothie

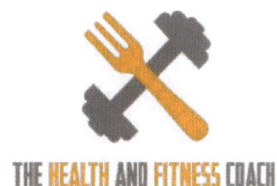

100g frozen mixed berries
100g frozen ripe banana
200ml unsweetened almond milk
juice of ½ lime
20g fresh spinach
25g vanilla flavour whey or rice protein powder (optional)

SERVES 1

Place all of the ingredients in a blender and blend until creamy. Serve.

Consume immediately.

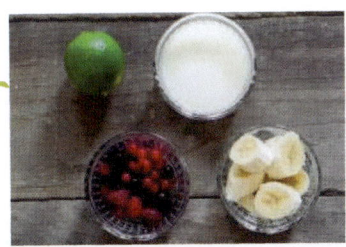

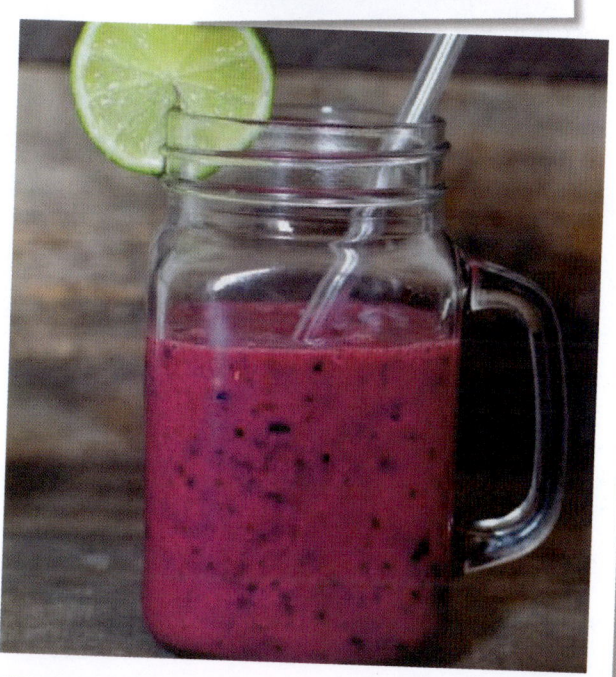

PER SERVING:
269 Calories
33g Carbs
23g Protein
5g Fat

https://thehealthandfitnesscoach.co.uk
DRINKS

Fruit & nut smoothie

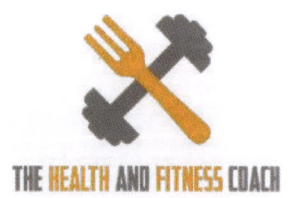

170ml unsweetened almond milk (or use milk of your choice)
50g frozen mango
1 kiwi fruit, peeled
25g vanilla flavour whey or rice protein powder (optional)
1 tsp vanilla extract
15g oats (use gluten free if preferred)
1 tsp flaxseed
4 walnut halves
3 ice cubes

SERVES 1

Place all of the ingredients in a blender and blend until creamy. Serve.

Consume immediately.

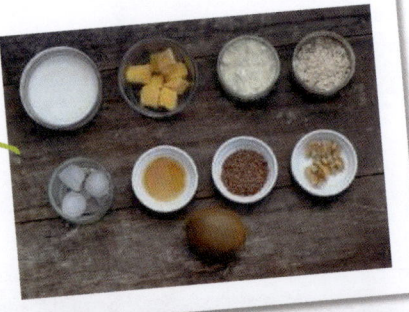

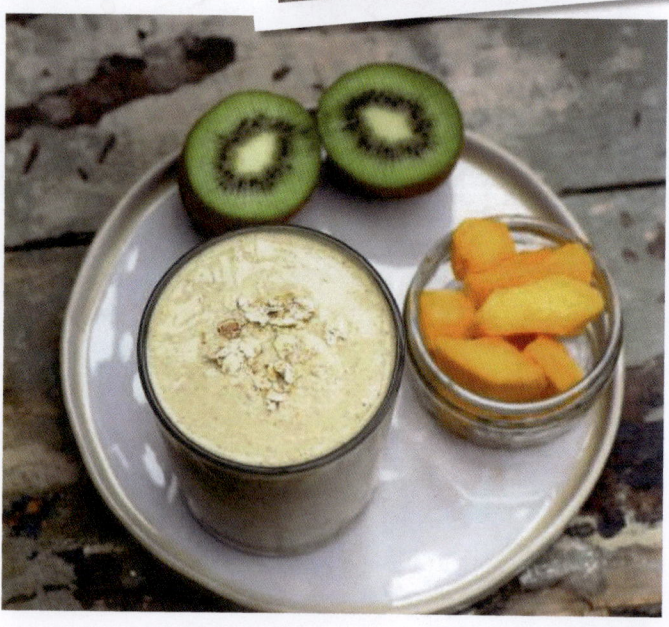

PER SERVING:
328 Calories
29g Carbs
26g Protein
12g Fat

https://thehealthandfitnesscoach.co.uk

Coconut dream smoothie

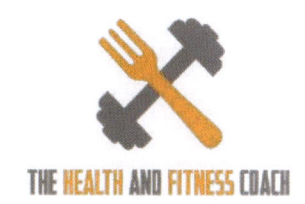

80ml tinned coconut milk
100ml unsweetened (long life) coconut drink or almond milk
1 tbsp unsweetened coconut flakes
30g vanilla or coconut flavour whey or rice protein powder (optional)
60g frozen banana
1 tsp flaxseed

SERVES 1

Place all of the ingredients in a blender and blend until creamy. Serve.

Consume immediately.

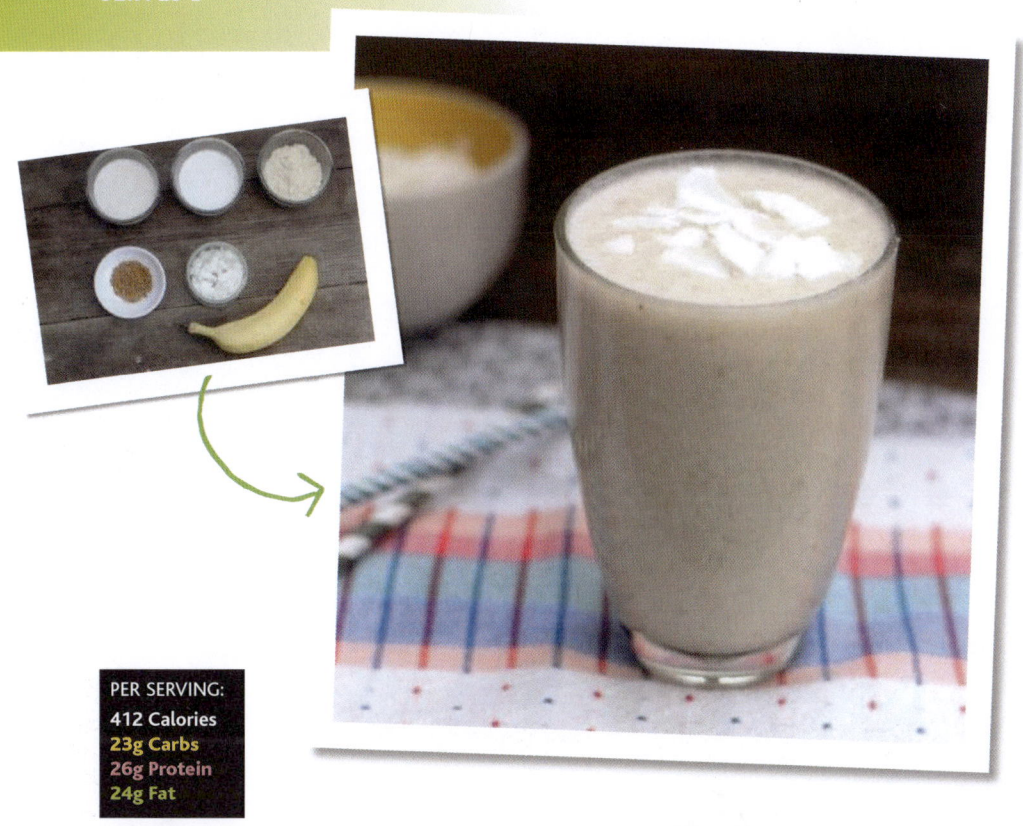

PER SERVING:
412 Calories
23g Carbs
26g Protein
24g Fat

https://thehealthandfitnesscoach.co.uk

DRINKS

Fruity frozen yoghurt

250g Greek yoghurt (use dairy free if preferred)
30g vanilla flavour whey or rice protein powder
a pinch of sea salt
120g frozen mango, pineapple or peach (or a mixture or each)

for the topping:
a sprinkle of freeze-dried pineapple or raspberries (optional)

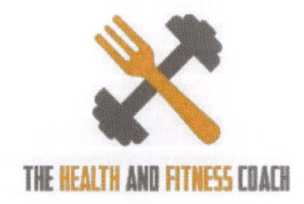

SERVES 2

Place all of the ingredients in a food processor. Blend well until smooth. Pause and scrape down the sides and blades during blending, if required.

Divide the mixture between two serving bowls. Top with the freeze-dried fruit (if using).

Consume immediately or freeze on same day. If freezing, allow 20 minutes before serving, to thaw.

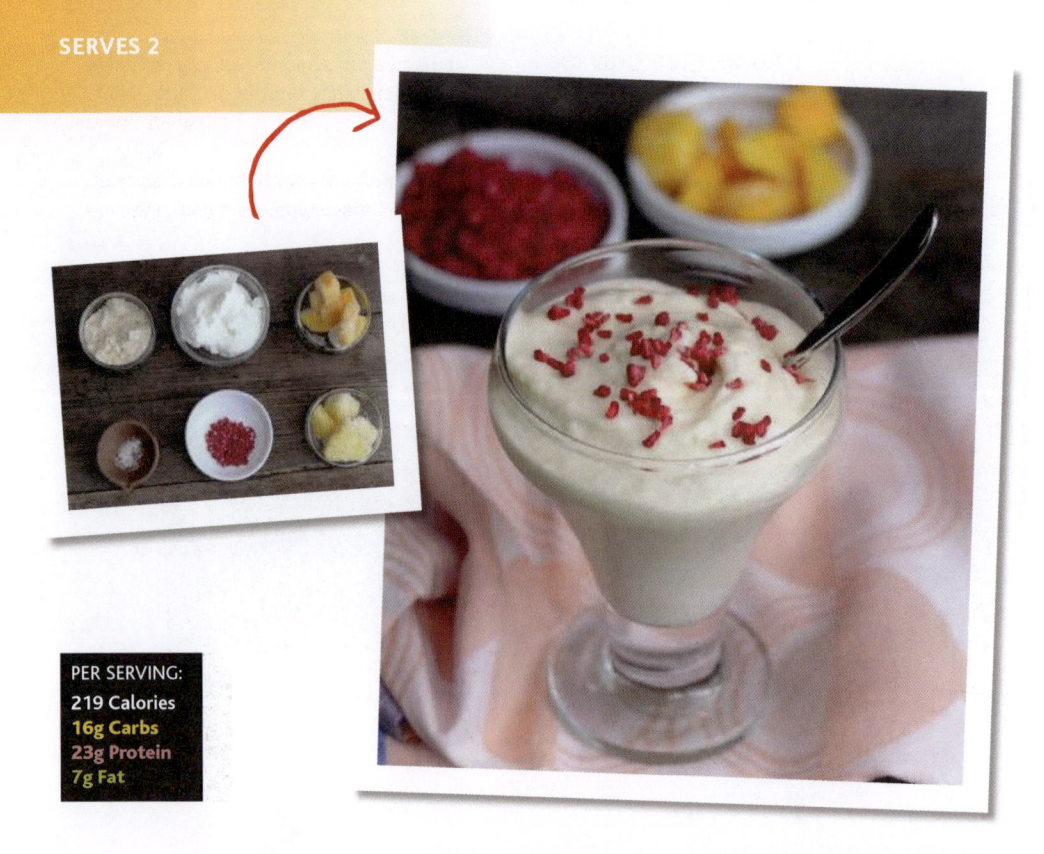

PER SERVING:
219 Calories
16g Carbs
23g Protein
7g Fat

https://thehealthandfitnesscoach.co.uk

SNACKS

Sticky pear & chocolate squares

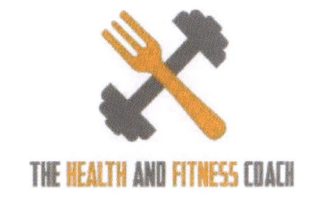

175g cooking apple, peeled, core removed and chopped
80g dark chocolate (minimum 75% cocoa)
40g coconut oil plus a little extra to grease tin
1 small ripe banana, mashed
30ml honey or maple syrup
125ml unsweetened almond milk or long-life coconut milk
150g plain flour (use gluten free if preferred)
15g cocoa powder
a small pinch of baking powder
a small pinch of sea salt
200g ripe pears, peeled, cored and finely chopped

SERVES 9

Place the apple in a small saucepan of water over a medium/high heat. Bring to a boil, then reduce heat and simmer gently for 3 minutes. Drain well and set aside.

Preheat oven to 180°C/350°F. Line the base of a 15x15cm square baking tin with baking paper and lightly grease the sides with coconut oil.

Place the dark chocolate and coconut oil in a small saucepan over a low heat. Heat gently, stirring occasionally until melted. Set aside. Place the mashed banana in a large bowl. Add the honey, milk, cooked apple and melted chocolate, and stir well.

Place the dry ingredients in a separate bowl and stir. Add the wet mixture to the dry mixture and stir thoroughly. Stir in the chopped pears. Bake for 35-40 minutes, or until a skewer inserted comes out clean. Allow to cool thoroughly in the tin. Cut into 9 pieces.

Store any leftovers in an airtight container and refrigerate for up to 2 days or freeze on same day.

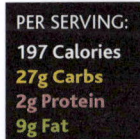

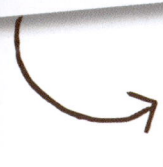

PER SERVING:
197 Calories
27g Carbs
2g Protein
9g Fat

https://thehealthandfitnesscoach.co.uk

SNACKS

Nutty marmalade bars

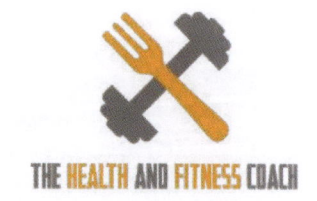

THE HEALTH AND FITNESS COACH

1 tsp melted coconut oil
100g almonds
100g unsalted roasted peanuts
20g pumpkin seeds
25g sunflower seeds
5g sesame seeds
a pinch of sea salt
for the syrup:
80g reduced sugar marmalade (or substitute with apricot jam)
3 tbsps maple syrup

MAKES 8 BARS

Preheat oven to 170°C/350°F. Line an oven tray with baking paper. Lightly brush the paper with melted coconut oil.

Place the nuts, seeds and salt in a large bowl.

Place the syrup ingredients in a saucepan over a medium heat. Bring to a boil then reduce heat to simmer. Heat, stirring for 3-4 minutes, or until the mixture has thickened slightly.

Immediately pour the hot syrup over the nuts and stir until well combined.

Transfer to the tray and spread evenly. Place a sheet of baking paper over the top and press down firmly to compact the mixture. Neaten up the sides using a spatula.

Bake for 30 minutes. Allow to cool then cut into 8 bars. The bars should harden as they cool.

Store in an airtight container for up to 1 week.

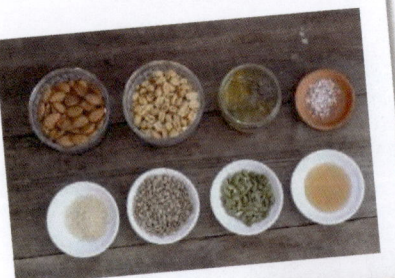

PER BAR:
223 Calories
14g Carbs
8g Protein
15g Fat

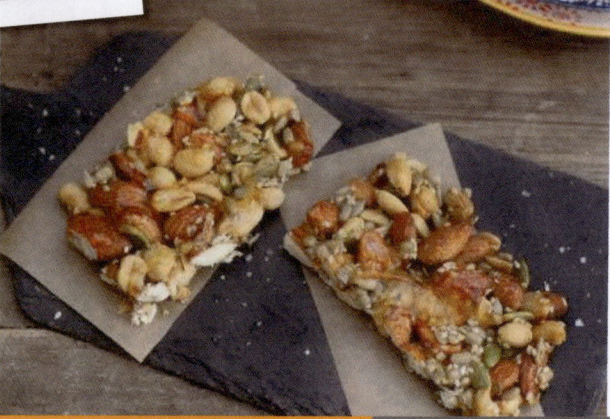

https://thehealthandfitnesscoach.co.uk

SNACKS   11

Passion fruit cheesecake

for the base:
70g soft pitted dates
170g walnuts
30g oats (use gluten free if preferred)
2 tbsps maple syrup

for the filling:
250g cream cheese (use dairy free if preferred)
140g Greek yoghurt (use dairy free if preferred)
1 egg
40g vanilla flavour whey or rice protein powder
the seeds of 2 passion fruit

for the topping (optional):
seeds of 1 passion fruit
60ml recently boiled water
1 tsp gelatine powder

SERVES 8

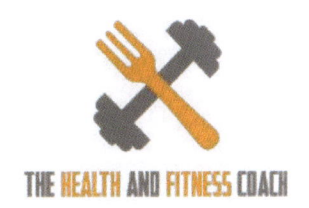

Preheat oven to 180°C/350°F. Line the base of an 18cm diameter round cake tin with baking paper.

Place the base ingredients in a blender or food processor and blend until finely ground. Transfer to the tin and press down firmly to compact.

Place the cream cheese, yoghurt, protein powder and egg in a large bowl. Blend well using an electric hand mixer, until all lumps are removed. Stir in the passion fruit seeds.

Pour the mixture over the base layer. Gently shake the tin from side to side, to distribute the topping evenly over the base. Bake for 15-20 minutes, or until the centre is still slightly soft. Allow to cool in the tin.

Stir the water and gelatine in a jug, until dissolved. Stir in the passion fruit seeds. Spread evenly over the cheesecake and refrigerate for 30 minutes, or until set.

Store any leftovers in an airtight container and refrigerate for up to 3 days or freeze on same day.

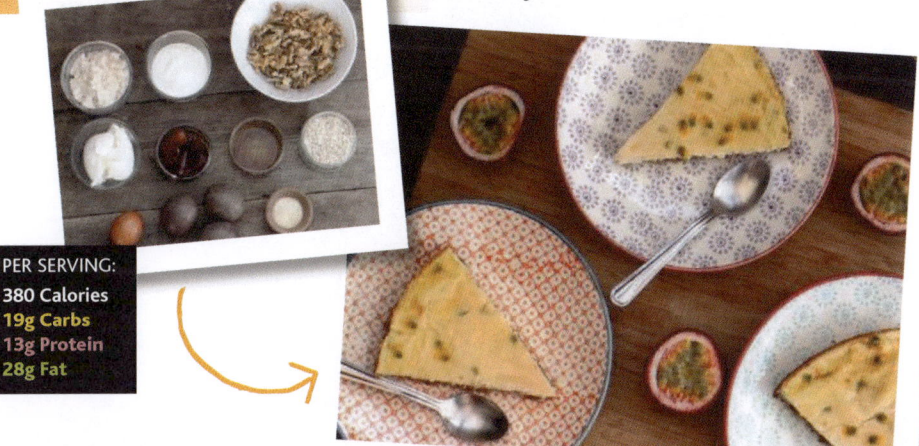

PER SERVING:
380 Calories
19g Carbs
13g Protein
28g Fat

https://thehealthandfitnesscoach.co.uk

Creamy coconut & cashew protein yoghurt

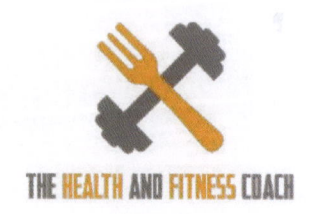

200g Greek yoghurt (use dairy free if preferred)
40g coconut cream (use the fat part from the top of a tin of coconut milk)
25g vanilla or coconut flavour whey or rice protein powder
1 tsp cashew butter
1 tsp vanilla extract or vanilla bean paste
50g frozen banana

for the topping:
a sprinkle of hemp or chia seeds
a drizzle of maple syrup (optional)
a sprinkle of cashew nuts, chopped

SERVES 2

Place all of the ingredients in a food processor or blender. Blend well until smooth.

Divide the mixture between two serving bowls. Add the toppings and serve.

Consume immediately

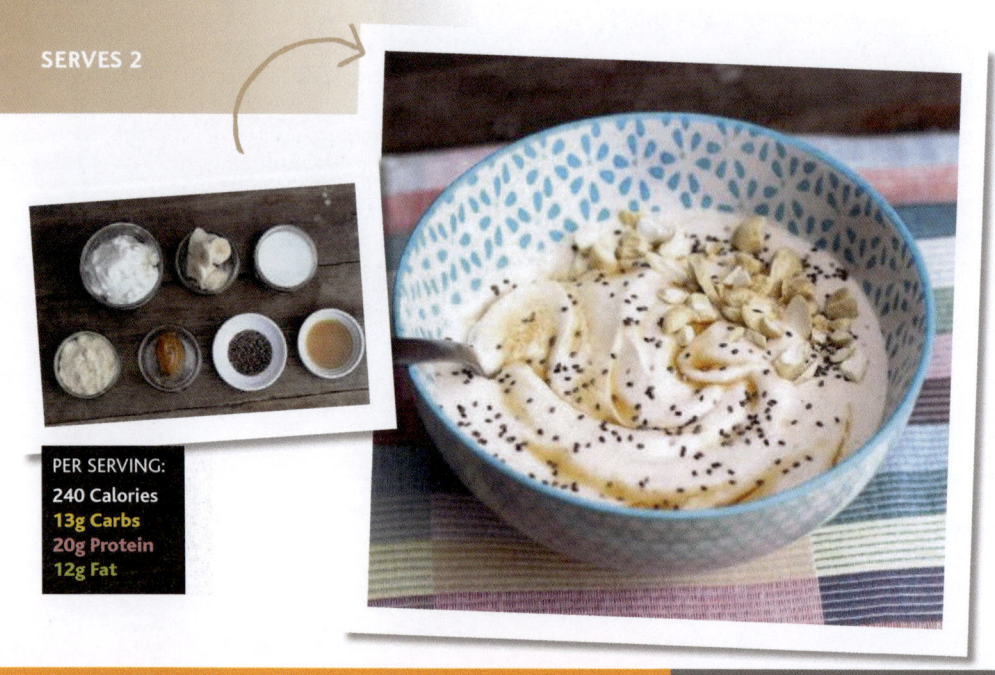

PER SERVING:
240 Calories
13g Carbs
20g Protein
12g Fat

SNACKS

No bake brownies

300g pitted Deglet nour or Medjool dates
90g ground almonds
3 tbsps cocoa powder
1 tsp vanilla extract
2 tbsps cold water
a small pinch of sea salt

MAKES 6 BROWNIES

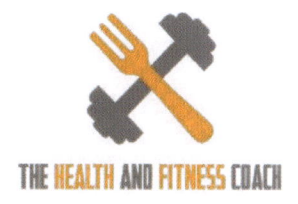

Line the base of a medium-sized loaf tin with baking paper.

Place the ingredients in a high speed blender or food processor. Process until a dough forms. Stop and scrape down the sides if necessary.

Transfer the dough to the tin and press down firmly, until the dough is evenly distributed over the base.

Refrigerate for 2 hours, or until firm. Cut into 6 pieces.

Store any leftovers in an airtight container and refrigerate for up to 4 days or freeze on same day.

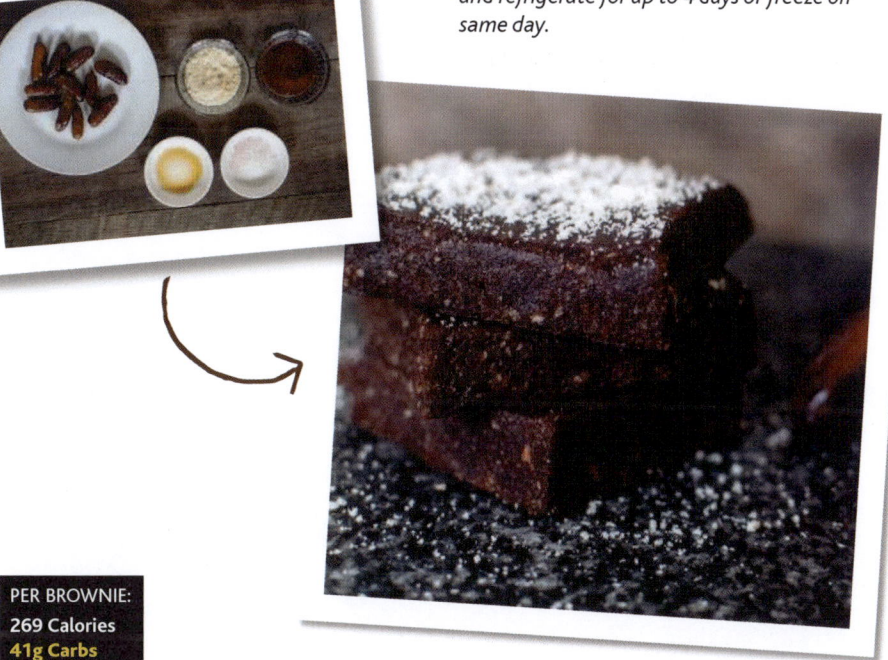

PER BROWNIE:
269 Calories
41g Carbs
6g Protein
9g Fat

https://thehealthandfitnesscoach.co.uk

Zesty chocolate fudge

65g coconut oil
40g cocoa powder
40g chocolate or vanilla whey or rice protein powder
30g dried fruit of your choice (pineapple, mango, apricots, cranberries, raisins, prunes etc), chopped
25g brazil nuts, almonds or cashews, chopped
3 tbsps maple syrup
1 tsp vanilla extract
½ tsp orange extract
a small pinch of sea salt
2 tbsps orange zest, finely grated

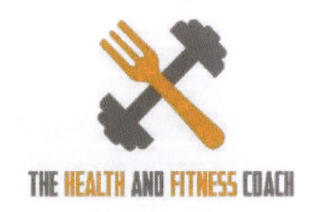

MAKES 16 PIECES

Line the base of a 15x15cm baking tin with baking paper.

Heat the coconut oil in a saucepan over a low heat until melted. Remove from the heat and whisk in the cocoa powder until smooth.

Whisk in the protein powder until smooth, then stir in the remaining ingredients, except for the zest.

Transfer the mixture into the tin, then sprinkle over the orange zest, pressing it gently onto the surface of the mixture.

Refrigerate for 1 hour, or until set. Cut into 16 pieces.

Store any leftovers in an airtight container and refrigerate for up to 5 days or freeze on same day.

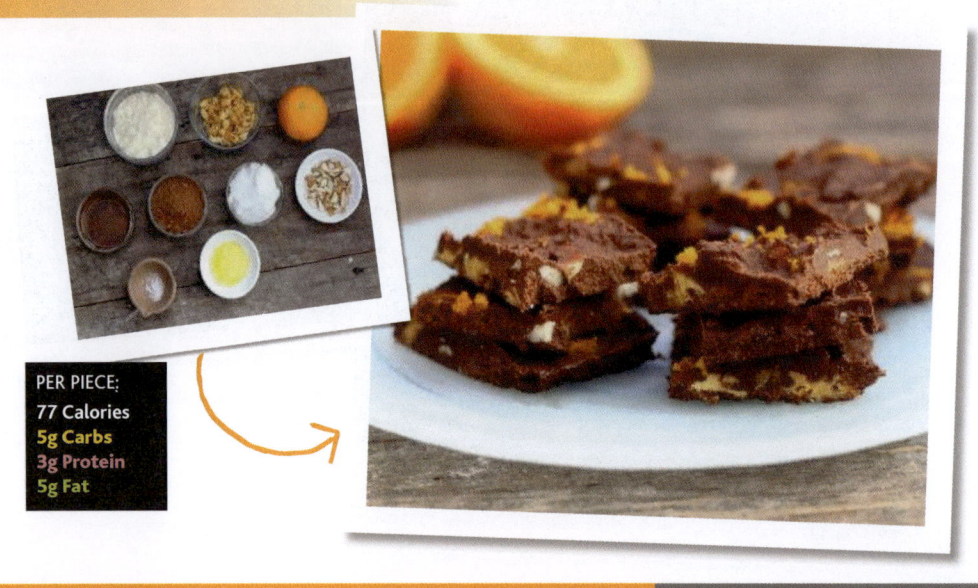

PER PIECE:
77 Calories
5g Carbs
3g Protein
5g Fat

https://thehealthandfitnesscoach.co.uk

SNACKS

Banana choc chip bars

3 medium-sized bananas, mashed
200g oats (use gluten free if preferred)
120g almond, cashew or peanut butter
30g banana or vanilla flavour whey or rice protein powder (optional)
20g dark chocolate (minimum 75% cocoa), cut into small chunks

MAKES 9 BARS

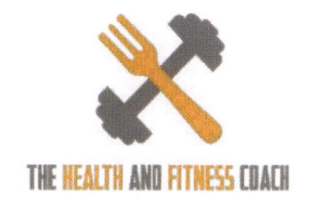

Preheat oven to 180°C/350°F. Line the base of a 15x15cm baking tin with baking paper.

Mash the banana in a large bowl. Add the remaining ingredients, except for the chocolate, and stir until thoroughly combined.

Stir in the chocolate chunks. Transfer the mixture into the tin and press down evenly with a spoon.

Bake for 15-20 minutes, or until golden on the outside and firm in the centre.

Allow to cool then cut into 9 bars.

Store any leftovers in an airtight container and refrigerate for up to 2 days or freeze on same day.

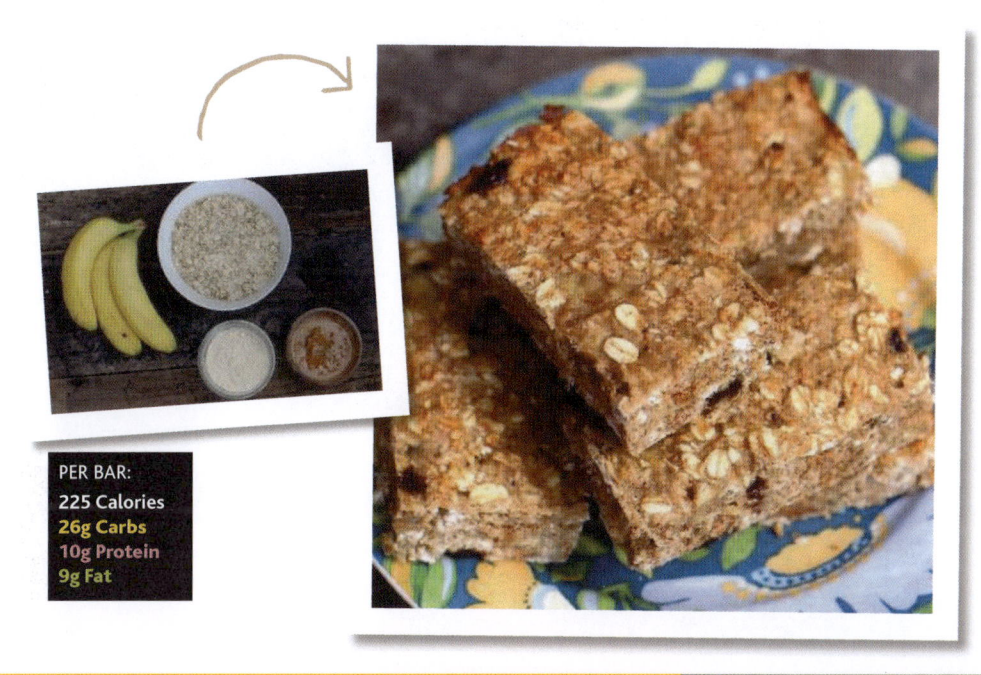

PER BAR:
225 Calories
26g Carbs
10g Protein
9g Fat

THE HEALTH AND FITNESS COACH

Oaty cookies

THE HEALTH AND FITNESS COACH

3 medium-sized ripe bananas
200g oats (use gluten free if preferred)
40g raisins
a sprinkle of ground cinnamon
1 tsp stevia (or use sweetener of your choice)
30g dark chocolate (minimum 70% cocoa), cut into chunks
25g hazelnuts

MAKES 8 COOKIES

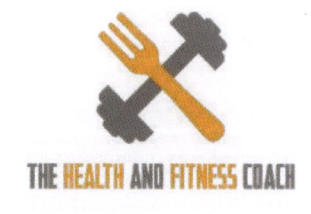

Preheat oven to 170°C/350°F. Line an oven tray with baking paper.

Mash the banana in a large bowl.

Add the remaining ingredients and stir until well combined.

Divide the mixture into 8 pieces and roll into balls. Place onto the tray, leaving a small gap between each ball. Gently flatten until around 2cm thickness.

Bake for 15 minutes or until firm. Allow to cool on the tray.

Store any leftovers in an airtight container for up to 4 days or freeze on same day.

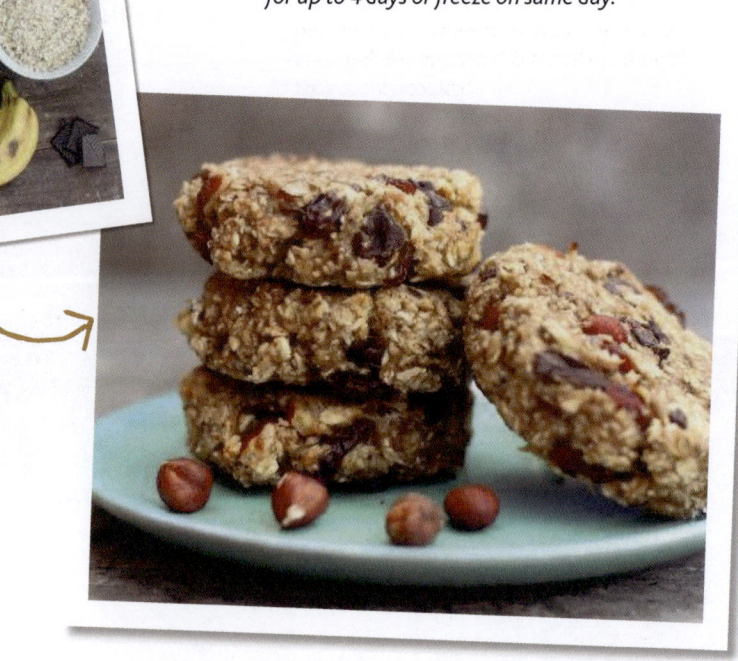

PER COOKIE:
198 Calories
31g Carbs
5g Protein
6g Fat

https://thehealthandfitnesscoach.co.uk

SNACKS

Peanut & coconut energy balls

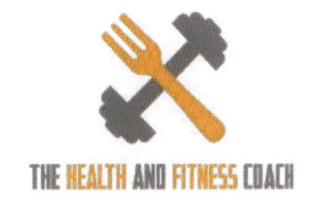

220g crunchy peanut butter
5 pitted Medjool or Deglet Nour dates
50g shelled hempseed
40g chia seeds
3 tbsps vanilla flavour whey or rice protein powder
5 tbsps desiccated coconut

MAKES 18 BALLS

Place the peanut butter, dates, hempseed, chia seeds and protein powder in a food processor. Blend well to form a dough.

Using a tablespoon, scoop out some of the mixture and roll into a ball.

Repeat step with the remaining mixture.

Roll the balls in desiccated coconut.

Freeze the balls for 25 minutes, or until firm. Serve.

Store any leftovers in an airtight container and refrigerate for up to one week or freeze on same day.

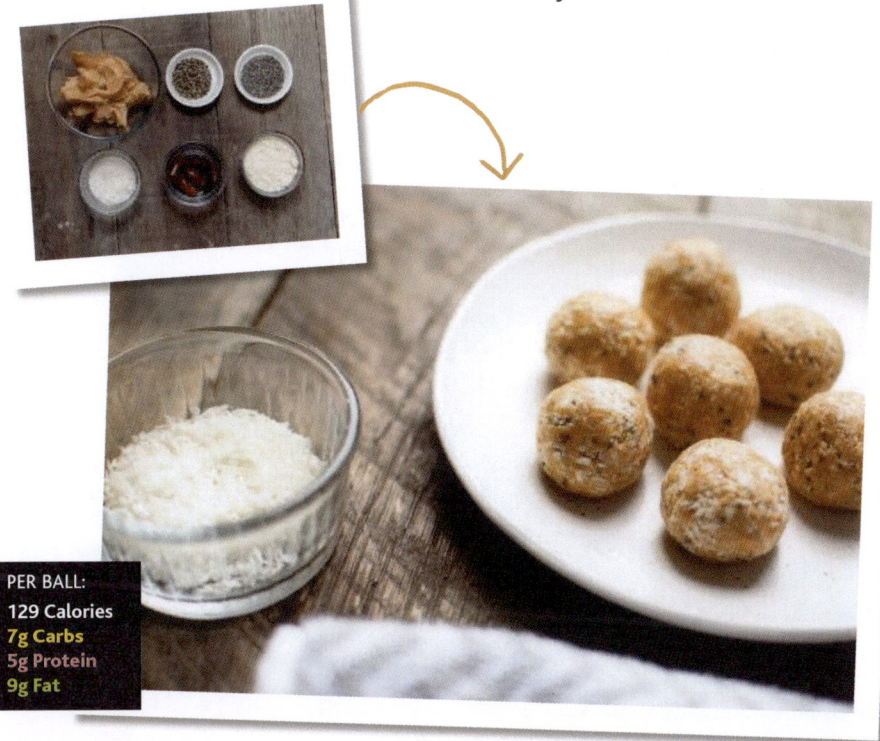

PER BALL:
129 Calories
7g Carbs
5g Protein
9g Fat

Beetroot, berry & chocolate cake

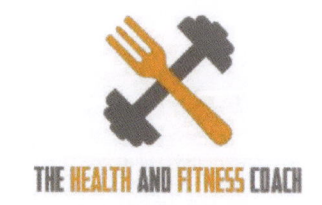

1 tsp butter or coconut oil, to grease cake tin
100g dark chocolate (minimum 70% cocoa)
3 tbsps butter
250g cooked beetroot, puréed
4 eggs
4 tbsps honey or maple syrup
3 tsps plain flour (or use gluten free flour of your choice)
2 tbsps cocoa powder
1 tsp baking powder
a pinch of sea salt
4 tsps desiccated coconut (optional)
125g ground almonds
100g fresh mixed berries (or use frozen - defrosted and at room temperature)

to decorate:
1 tsp cocoa powder
a few mixed berries

SERVES 10

Preheat oven to 180°C/350°F. Lightly grease the base and sides of a 9 inch cake tin with butter / coconut oil. Line the base with baking paper.

Place the chocolate and butter in a heatproof bowl. Pour several inches of boiling water into a shallow wide-based dish. Place over a medium heat and allow the water to simmer gently. Place the bowl of chocolate and butter into the shallow dish of water and heat until melted, stirring continuously. Remove from heat and set aside.

Place the puréed beetroot and remaining ingredients in a large bowl. Blend well using an electric hand mixer.

Pour the mixture into the cake tin. Bake for 20-25 minutes. A skewer inserted into the centre of the cake will come out clean when cooked. Remove from tin and transfer to a wire rack until cooled completely.

Lightly dust the top of the cake with cocoa powder. Serve with berries.

Store any leftovers in an airtight container for up to 4 days or freeze on same day.

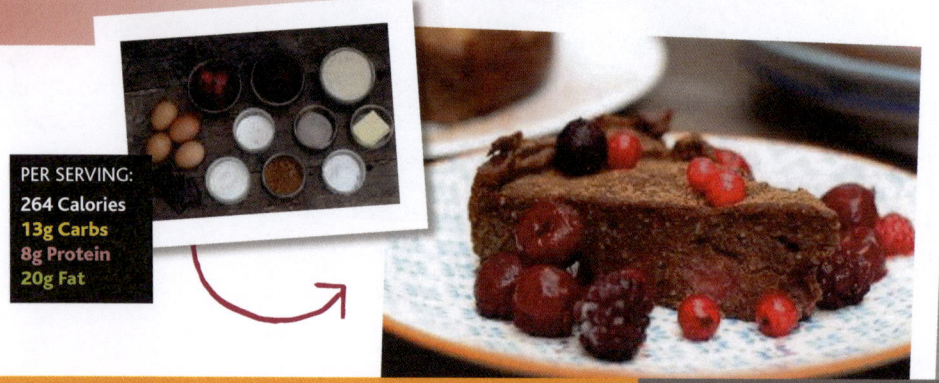

PER SERVING:
264 Calories
13g Carbs
8g Protein
20g Fat

https://thehealthandfitnesscoach.co.uk

SNACKS 19

Peanut butter, chocolate & banana ice cream

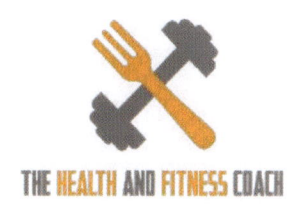

THE HEALTH AND FITNESS COACH

4 medium-sized ripe bananas
50g vanilla flavour whey or rice protein powder
80g crunchy peanut butter
30g dark chocolate or milk chocolate, cut into chunks

SERVES 3

Place the bananas and protein powder in a food processor. Blend well until smooth.

Add the peanut butter and pulse briefly to combine.

Stir in the chocolate chunks.

Transfer to a sealable airtight container and freeze for one hour. Stir well and freeze for one hour or until firm. Serve.

Store any leftovers in an airtight container and freeze for up to 3 weeks.

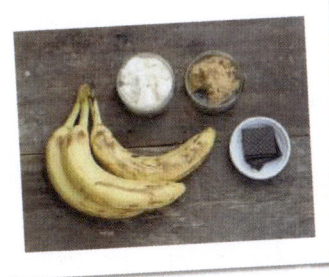

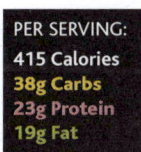

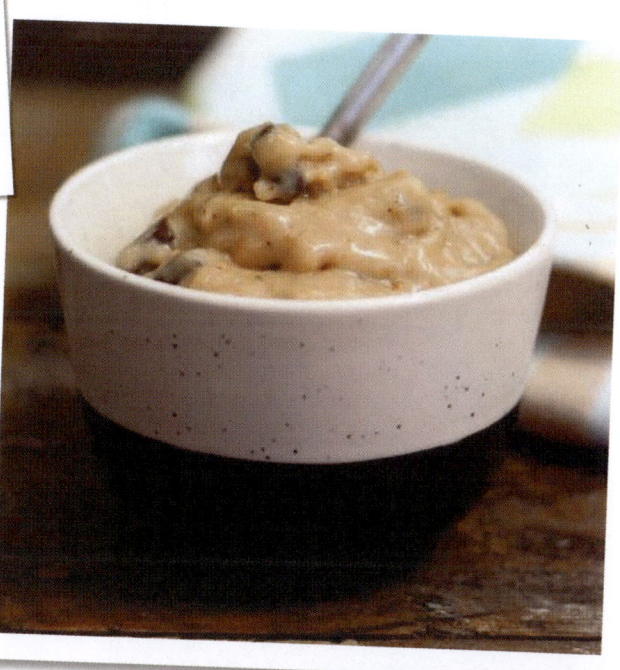

PER SERVING:
415 Calories
38g Carbs
23g Protein
19g Fat

https://thehealthandfitnesscoach.co.uk

SNACKS 20

Apple oaty bars

2 small ripe bananas
200g oats (use gluten free if preferred)
1 tsp ground cinnamon
1 sweet apple, cored and chopped finely
60g butter or coconut oil, melted
30g honey or maple syrup
60g raisins
30g dark chocolate (minimum 70% cocoa), cut into chunks

MAKES 8 BARS

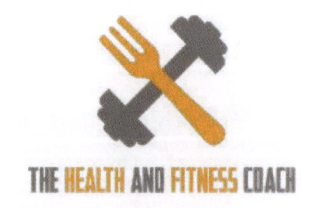

Preheat oven to 180°C/350°F. Lightly grease the base and sides of a 15x15cm square tin with coconut oil. Line the base with baking paper.

Mash the bananas in a large bowl, until smooth.

Add the oats, cinnamon, apple, melted butter/oil and honey. Mix well until thoroughly combined.

Stir in the raisins and dark chocolate.

Transfer the mixture to the tin. Bake for 20-25 minutes, or until golden.

Cut into 8 bars.

Store any leftovers in an airtight container for up to 3 days.

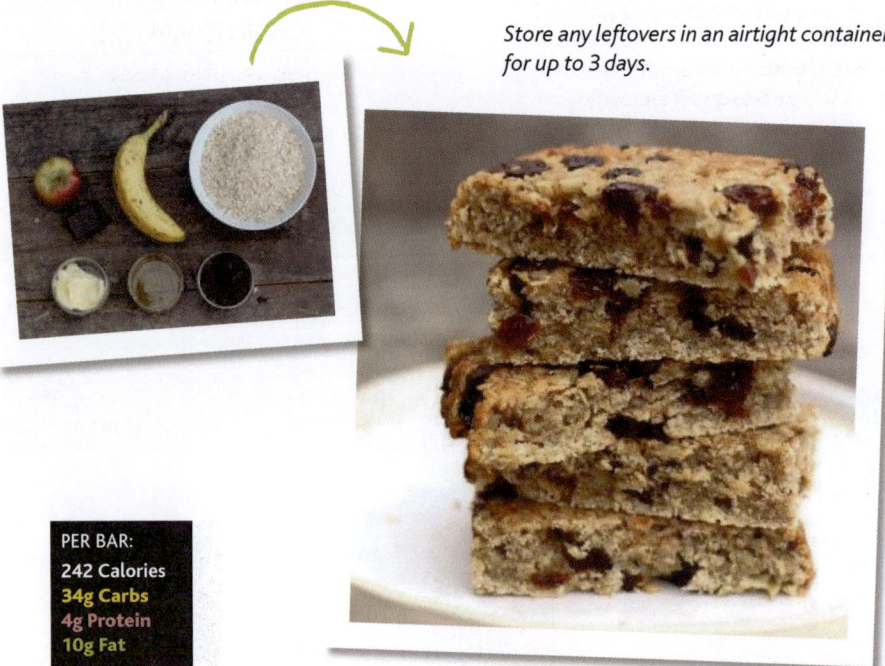

PER BAR:
242 Calories
34g Carbs
4g Protein
10g Fat

https://thehealthandfitnesscoach.co.uk

SNACKS   21

Coconut bliss energy balls

for the energy balls:
90g desiccated coconut
30g vanilla flavour whey or rice protein powder
50g ground almonds
30g oats (use gluten free if preferred)
40g coconut oil, melted
2 tbsps maple syrup or honey
2 tbsps unsweetened coconut milk
25g white chocolate (use a good quality Swiss chocolate), cut into small chunks (optional)

for the coating:
20g desiccated coconut

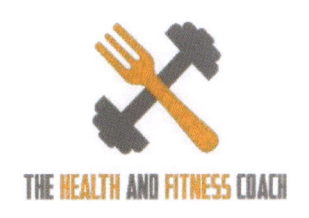

MAKES 10 ENERGY BALLS

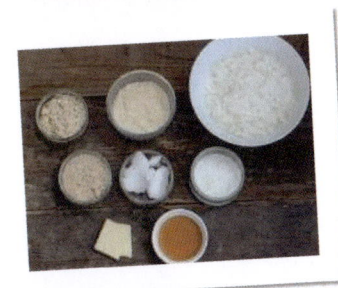

Place the energy ball ingredients into a high speed blender or food processor and blend until well combined. The mixture should be slightly sticky. Add more coconut milk if required.

Roll into 10 balls.

Sprinkle the desiccated coconut onto a plate. Roll each ball in the coconut.

Refrigerate for one hour then serve.

Store any leftovers in an airtight container and refrigerate for up to 3 days or freeze on same day.

PER BALL:
121 Calories
6g Carbs
4g Protein
9g Fat

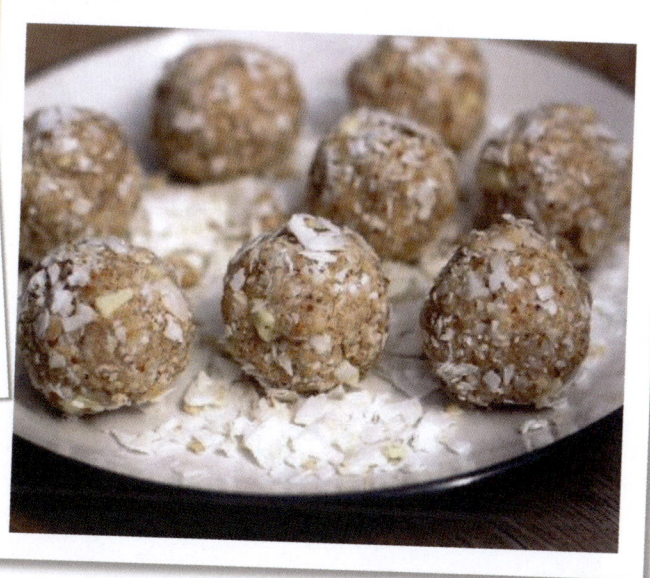

THE HEALTH AND FITNESS COACH

https://thehealthandfitnesscoach.co.uk

SNACKS

Berry banana smoothie bowl

100g frozen berries
½ a small frozen banana
30ml unsweetened almond milk
25g vanilla flavour whey or rice protein powder (optional)
a handful of fresh spinach leaves
for the toppings:
1 tbsp flaked almonds
1 tbsp sunflower, pumpkin or chia seeds

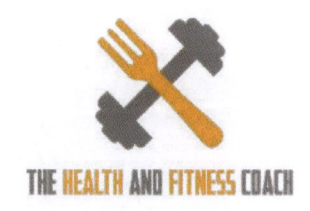

SERVES 1

Place the ingredients in a blender and blend well until smooth. Transfer to a serving bowl.

Add the toppings and serve.

Consume immediately.

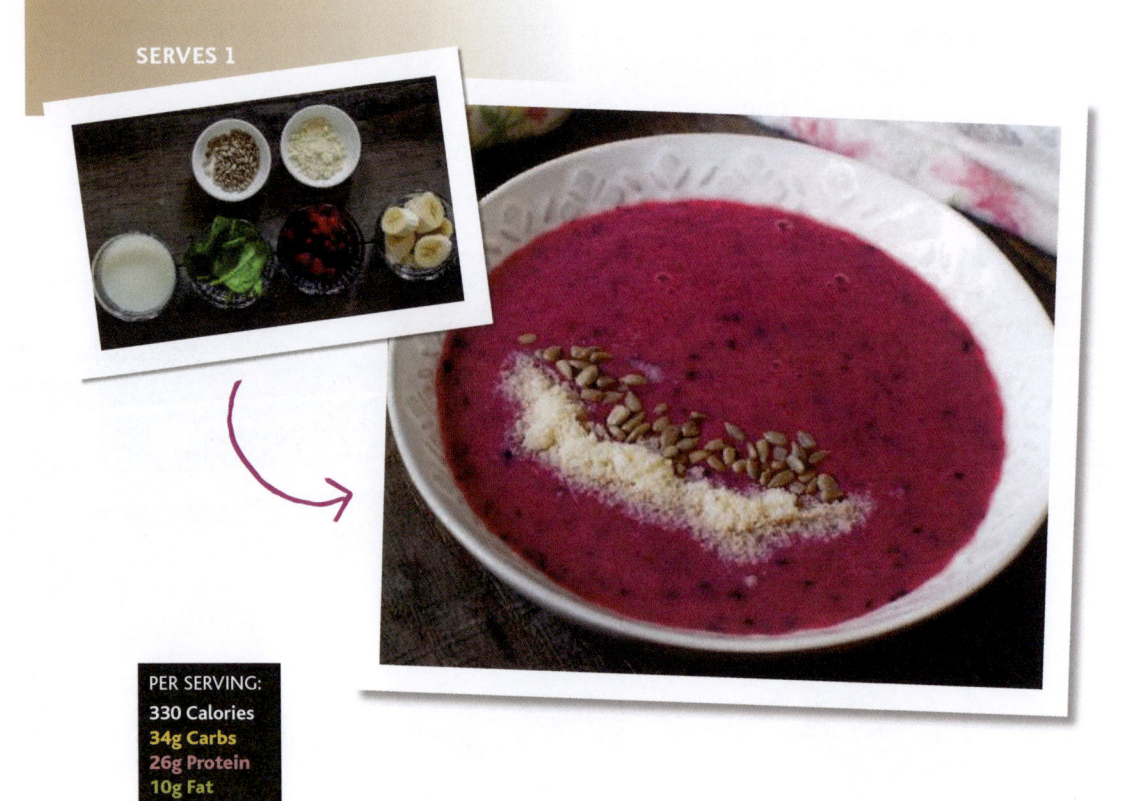

PER SERVING:
330 Calories
34g Carbs
26g Protein
10g Fat

https://thehealthandfitnesscoach.co.uk

BREAKFAST 23

Egg breakfast burrito

150g chicken breast
½ tsp sea salt
1 tsp ground black pepper
2 large eggs
1 tbsp whole milk or unsweetened almond milk
1 tbsp fresh parsley, finely chopped
a small pinch of sea salt
a pinch of ground black pepper
1 tsp butter or coconut oil
100g tinned black beans (drained weight)
1 small ripe avocado, finely sliced
50g Cheddar cheese, grated (use dairy free if preferred)

SERVES 2

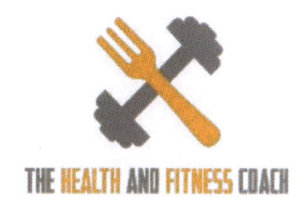

Place the chicken breast into a large saucepan. Season with salt and pepper. Cover with 1 inch of cold water.

Place the saucepan over a medium/high heat and bring the water to a boil. Reduce heat and simmer for 10 minutes, or until the chicken is thoroughly cooked.

Remove the chicken from the water and transfer to a plate to cool. Shred with a fork.

Whisk the eggs, milk, parsley, salt and pepper in a jug.

Melt the coconut oil in a large frying pan or skillet over a medium heat. Tilt the pan to coat the base then add the egg mixture. Tilt the pan to ensure the egg covers the entire base of the pan, then cook for 2 minutes.

Carefully flip or turn using a slice and cook for 2 minutes. Transfer to a plate and top with cheese, black beans, avocado and chicken. Roll up into a burrito. Cut in half and serve.

Store any leftovers in an airtight container and refrigerate for up to 1 day.

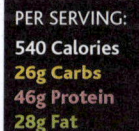

PER SERVING:
540 Calories
26g Carbs
46g Protein
28g Fat

https://thehealthandfitnesscoach.co.uk

BREAKFAST   24

Oaty power bowl

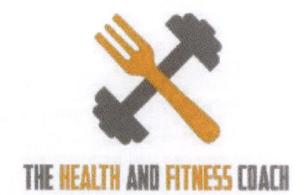

5g unsweetened coconut flakes
50g ripe banana, mashed
2 heaped tbsps chia seeds
35g oats (use gluten free if preferred)
a pinch of ground cinnamon
160ml unsweetened almond milk
90ml cold water

for the topping:
1 tsp ground flaxseed
5g almonds, chopped
½ tsp sunflower seeds
a sprinkle of ground cinnamon
a sprinkle of ground allspice (optional)
a sprinkle of dried cranberries

SERVES 1

Place the coconut flakes in a frying pan over a medium heat. Toast gently for 2-3 minutes, until the edges of the flakes just start to colour. Remove pan from heat and set aside.

Place the mashed banana, chia seeds, oats, cinnamon, almond milk and water in a saucepan. Place the saucepan over a medium heat and cook, stirring frequently for 5 minutes, or until thickened. Add more water during cooking time, if the mixture becomes too thick.

Transfer to a bowl and add the toasted coconut and toppings. Serve.

Consume immediately.

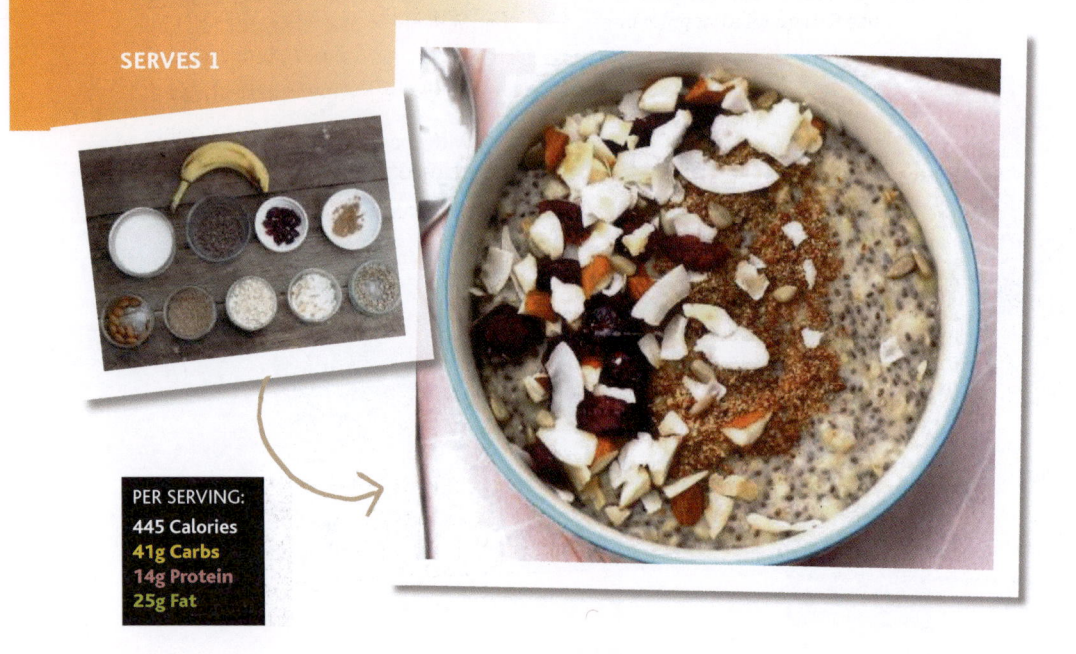

PER SERVING:
445 Calories
41g Carbs
14g Protein
25g Fat

Sweetcorn fritters topped with a poached egg

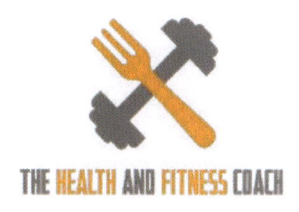

2 tbsps coconut oil
1 egg (per person)
¼ of a medium-sized ripe avocado (per person), sliced
1 tbsp fresh coriander, finely chopped

for the fritters:
65g rice flour or chickpea flour
80ml whole milk or unsweetened almond milk
180g (drained weight) tinned sweetcorn
3 spring onions, finely chopped
50g Cheddar cheese, grated
a pinch of sea salt and ground black pepper
2 eggs
¾ tsp curry powder

MAKES 9 FRITTERS

Mix the flour and milk in a large bowl with a balloon whisk, until thoroughly combined. Add the eggs and whisk lightly. Add the remaining fritter ingredients and mix well.

Melt half of the oil in a large frying pan over a medium heat. Place spoonfuls of the mixture into the pan, 1 tbsp at a time, leaving a gap around each one.

Fry gently for 2-4 minutes, or until the underside is golden. Turn and cook for 3 minutes on the other side, or until golden. Transfer the fritters to a plate. Repeat with the remaining oil and batter.

Bring a small saucepan of water to the boil. Reduce heat to simmer gently. Carefully crack one egg into a ladle. Pour the egg into the water. Repeat with remaining eggs. Allow to cook for around 3-4 minutes then remove with a slotted spoon, draining off any excess water. Serve with the avocado.

Store any leftover fritters in an airtight container and refrigerate for up to 2 days or freeze on same day.

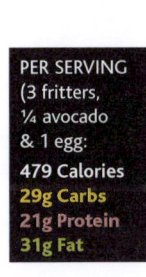

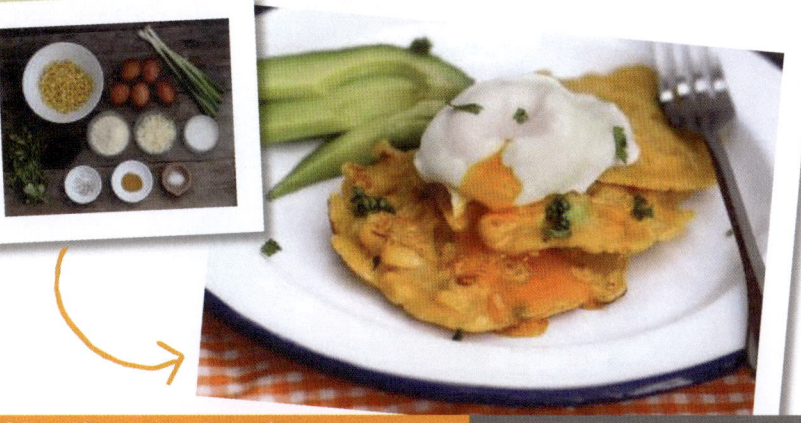

PER SERVING
(3 fritters, ¼ avocado & 1 egg:
479 Calories
29g Carbs
21g Protein
31g Fat

THE HEALTH AND FITNESS COACH

https://thehealthandfitnesscoach.co.uk

BREAKFAST

Quick & easy protein pancakes

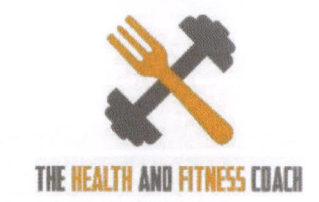

1 tbsp coconut oil

for the pancakes:
2 eggs
40g vanilla flavour whey or rice protein powder
½ tsp baking powder
60ml unsweetened almond milk

SERVES 2

Place the pancake ingredients in a blender and blend well until smooth. Heat ½ tsp coconut oil in a large frying pan over a medium heat.

When the oil is hot, pour around a quarter of the batter into the frying pan.

When bubbles start to form on the top of the pancake, turn or flip the pancake.

Cook for another 1-2 minutes. Transfer to a plate. Repeat steps with the remaining oil and batter. Serve.

Consume immediately.

Serving suggestion:

Drizzle lightly with honey or maple syrup and serve with fresh berries of your choice

PER SERVING:
213 Calories
2g Carbs
22g Protein
13g Fat

https://thehealthandfitnesscoach.co.uk   BREAKFAST   27

Veggie-rich bake

THE HEALTH AND FITNESS COACH

1 tsp coconut oil, for frying (plus a little extra to grease dish)
a small red onion, cut into thin wedges
a handful of Tenderstem broccoli, trimmed
1 red or yellow bell-pepper, deseeded and diced
8 eggs plus 2 egg whites
1 tbsp Parmesan, grated (use dairy free cheese if preferred)
a few fresh basil or parsley leaves, finely chopped
a pinch of sea salt and ground black pepper
1 medium-sized ripe avocado

SERVES 4

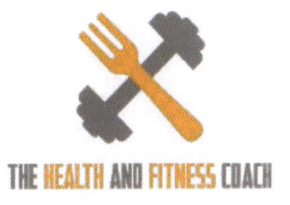

Preheat oven to 175°C/350°F. Lightly grease an ovenproof dish with coconut oil.

Heat the oil in a frying pan over a medium heat. Add the onion and sauté for 4-5 minutes, stirring occasionally until soft.

Add the bell-pepper and broccoli and fry gently for 4-5 minutes, stirring occasionally. Transfer to the dish.

Crack the eggs and egg whites into a large jug. Beat gently with a fork. Add the cheese, fresh herbs, salt and pepper and stir.

Peel the avocado, remove the stone and chop. Distribute evenly over the vegetables.

Pour the egg mixture over the top, to cover the vegetables.

Bake for 20 minutes or until the centre is cooked. Cut into 4 pieces. Serve.

Store any leftovers in an airtight container and refrigerate for up to 3 days.

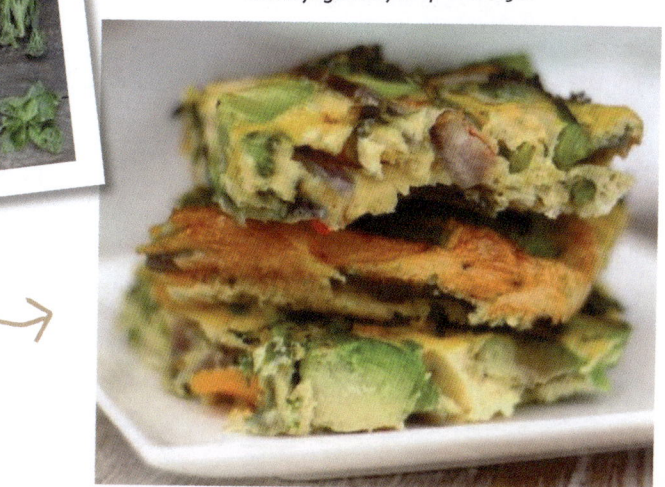

PER SERVING:
232 Calories
6g Carbs
16g Protein
16g Fat

https://thehealthandfitnesscoach.co.uk

BREAKFAST

Breakfast bowl

2 eggs
3 tsps coconut oil
2 garlic cloves, peeled and minced
50g closed cup or button mushrooms, sliced
¼ tsp dried mixed herbs
a small pinch of paprika
¼ tsp allspice
a small pinch of sea salt
2 ripe salad tomatoes, cut into quarters
80g fresh spinach leaves
1 small white potato, peeled and cut into ½ inch thick cubes

SERVES 2

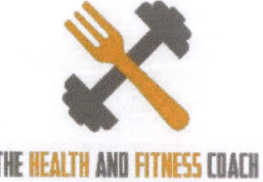

Fill a small saucepan with water and bring to a boil. Reduce the heat to low / medium and add the eggs. Cook for 10 minutes. Transfer the eggs to a bowl using a slotted spoon and allow to cool. Set aside the saucepan of water for later. Peel and slice or chop the eggs. Season with the salt and paprika.

Heat 1 tsp coconut oil in a large frying pan over a medium heat. Add the garlic, mushrooms, mixed herbs, paprika, allspice and salt. Fry gently, stirring occasionally for 5 minutes, or until the mushrooms have softened. Add the tomatoes and spinach, and cook for 3 minutes, stirring occasionally.

Place the saucepan of water back over a high heat and bring to the boil. Add the potatoes and cook for 6-8 minutes or until fork tender. Drain well.

Heat the remaining oil in the frying pan and place over a medium heat. Add the potatoes and season with salt and pepper, if desired. Fry for 3 minutes, or until golden. Arrange the eggs, vegetables and potato in two serving bowls.

Consume immediately.

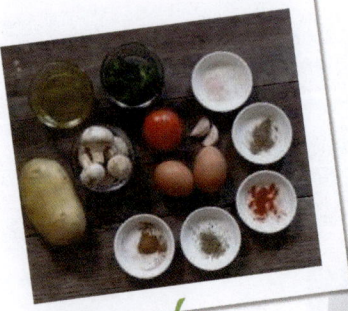

PER SERVING:
224 Calories
19g Carbs
10g Protein
12g Fat

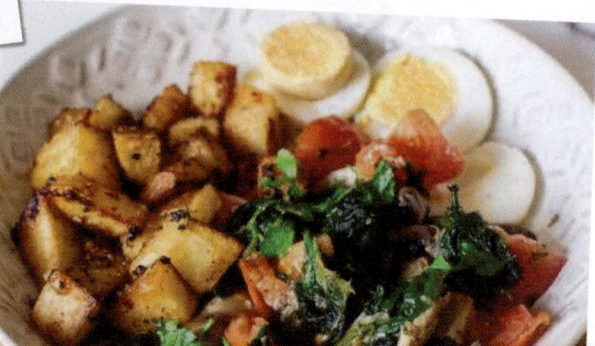

Strawberry & almond overnight oats

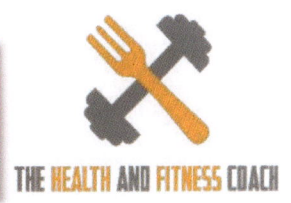

50g oats (use gluten free if preferred)
120ml unsweetened almond milk (or use milk of your choice)
30g Greek yoghurt (use dairy free if preferred)
½ tsp vanilla extract
60g frozen or fresh strawberries (if using fresh strawberries add them just before serving)
1 tbsp chia seeds
1 tsp honey or maple syrup
to serve:
1 tbsp flaked almonds

SERVES 1

Mix all of the ingredients in a sealable container. Stir well.

Cover and refrigerate overnight.

Transfer to a serving bowl and garnish with the flaked almonds. Serve.

Store any leftovers in an airtight container and refrigerate for up to 1 day.

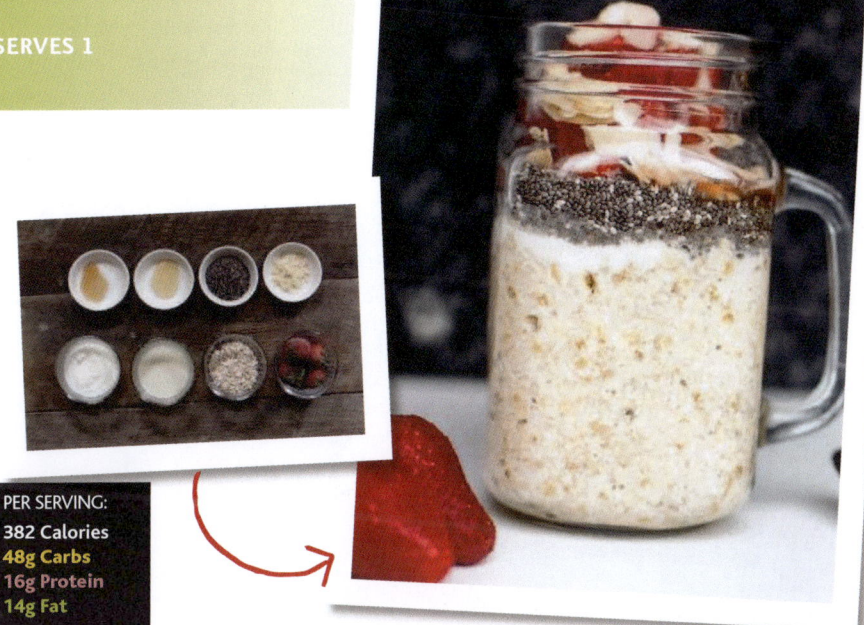

PER SERVING:
382 Calories
48g Carbs
16g Protein
14g Fat

BREAKFAST

Baked oat cups

½ tsp coconut oil (plus extra to grease muffin tin)
240ml unsweetened almond milk (or use milk of your choice)
2 large eggs
50g maple syrup
1 tsp vanilla extract
260g apples, peeled, cored and finely chopped
300g oats (use gluten free if preferred)
1 tsp baking powder
2 tsps ground cinnamon
½ tsp ground nutmeg
¼ tsp sea salt

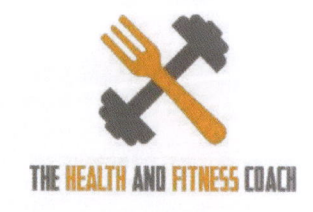

MAKES 12 CUPS

Preheat oven to 180C/350°F. Lightly grease 12 compartments of a muffin tin with coconut oil, or prepare a silicon muffin tray.

Pour the milk into a large jug. Add the eggs, maple syrup and vanilla extract. Whisk with a fork until combined.

Stir in the chopped apple.

Add the remaining ingredients and stir until well combined.

Spoon the mixture into the muffin tin compartments. Bake for 20-25 minutes or until a light golden brown and firm in the centre.

Leave to cool in the tin for 10 minutes. Transfer to a wire rack and allow to cool completely.

Store any leftovers in an airtight container and refrigerate for up to 3 days or freeze on same day.

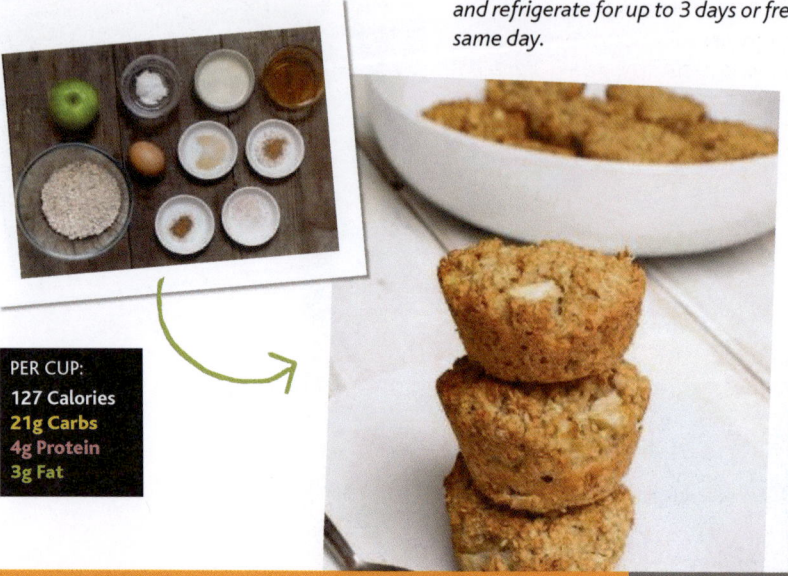

PER CUP:
127 Calories
21g Carbs
4g Protein
3g Fat

THE HEALTH AND FITNESS COACH

https://thehealthandfitnesscoach.co.uk

BREAKFAST 31

Sweetcorn, spinach & chive muffins

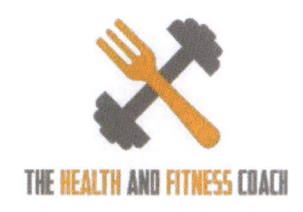

a small amount of butter or coconut oil to grease tin
100g button mushrooms, finely chopped
100g tinned sweetcorn, drained
a small handful of fresh spinach leaves, finely chopped
100g vine-ripened tomatoes, chopped
a pinch of sea salt and ground black pepper
a pinch of ground cumin
5 eggs
2 egg whites
50g Cheddar cheese, grated or Feta cheese, crumbled
1-2 tbsps fresh chives, finely chopped

MAKES 9 MUFFINS

Preheat oven to 180°C/350°F. Lightly grease 9 muffins tin compartments or prepare a large silicon muffin tin.

Place all of the ingredients in a large bowl and mix until combined.

Divide the mixture between the muffin tin compartments.

Bake for 20-25 minutes or until firm in the centre.

Allow to cool in the tin. Enjoy warm or cold.

Store any leftovers in an airtight container and refrigerate for 3 days.

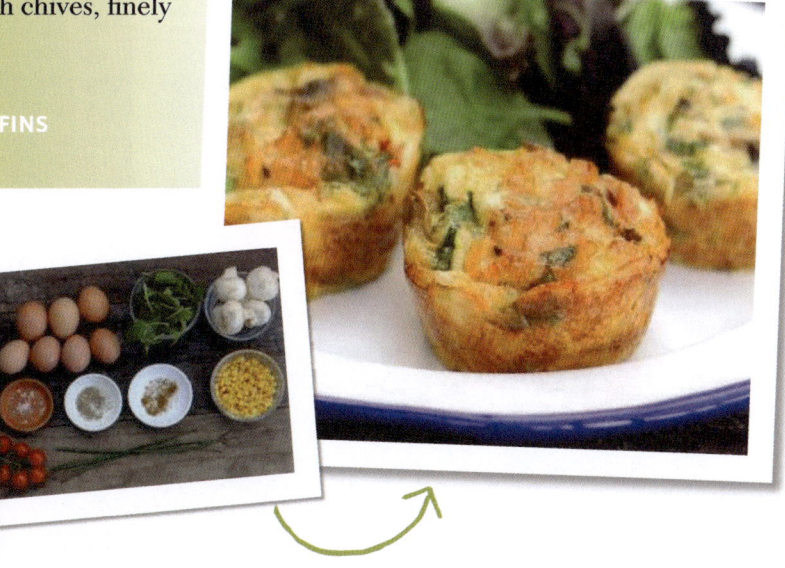

PER MUFFIN:
77 Calories
2g Carbs
6g Protein
5g Fat

https://thehealthandfitnesscoach.co.uk

BREAKFAST

Breakfast roasted peppers with eggs

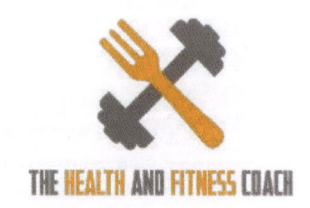

1 tbsp coconut oil
½ a medium-sized white onion, finely chopped
1 garlic clove, minced
200g tinned chopped tomatoes
125ml cold water
½ tsp sea salt
½ tsp ground black pepper
½ tsp dried mixed herbs
4 bell-peppers, tops and cores removed
50g Cheddar cheese, grated (use dairy free if preferred)
4 eggs

SERVES 2

Preheat oven to 180°C/350°F. Prepare a medium-sized ovenproof dish.

Heat the oil in a saucepan over a medium heat. Add the onion and sauté for 6-8 minutes, stirring occasionally until soft and translucent.

Add the garlic and fry gently for 3 minutes, stirring occasionally.

Add the chopped tomatoes, water, salt, pepper, and mixed herbs. Cook for 3 minutes then remove from the heat. Allow to cool for 5 minutes.

Using a hand blender, blend the sauce until smooth.

Stand the peppers upright in the dish. Stuff the cheese into each pepper, then pour the sauce around the base of the peppers.

Crack an egg into each pepper. Bake for 15 minutes, or until the eggs are cooked.

Consume immediately.

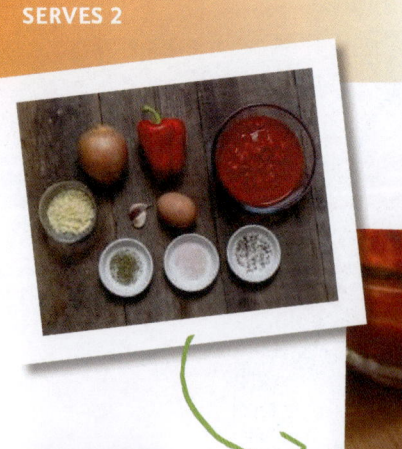

PER SERVING:
398 Calories
19g Carbs
22g Protein
26g Fat

https://thehealthandfitnesscoach.co.uk

BREAKFAST

Mango & berry smoothie bowl

50g frozen mango chunks
100g frozen blueberries or mixed berries
25g vanilla flavour whey or rice protein powder
160ml unsweetened almond milk
for the toppings:
20g chia seeds
40g berries of your choice

SERVES 1

Place the mango, berries, protein powder and 80ml milk in a blender and blend well until smooth.

Add the remaining milk a little at a time, until desired consistency is achieved.

Transfer the mixture to a bowl and add the toppings. Serve.

Consume immediately.

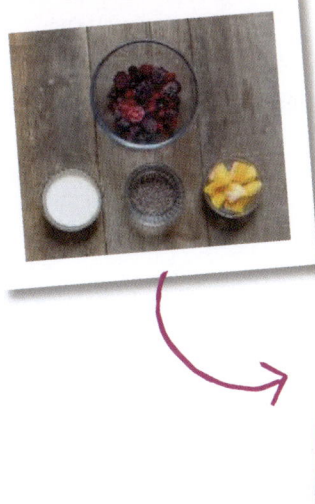

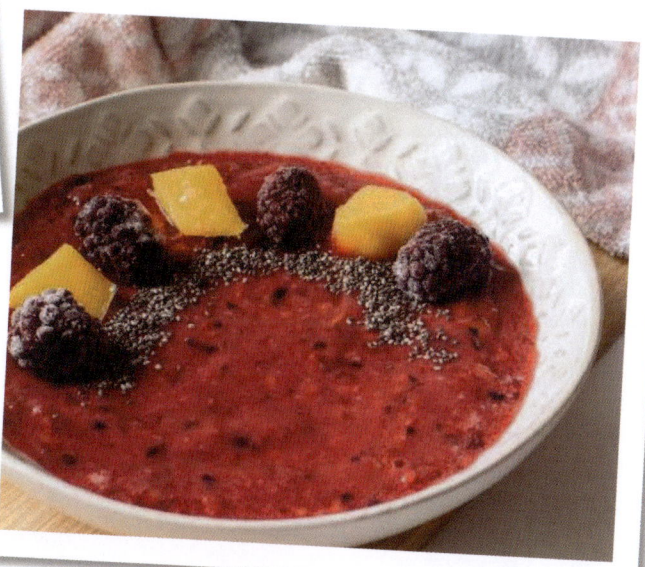

PER SERVING:
394 Calories
41g Carbs
26g Protein
14g Fat

https://thehealthandfitnesscoach.co.uk

Matcha smoothie bowl

for the smoothie bowl:
1 small ripe banana
1 tsp matcha powder
½ tsp honey or agave nectar
½ a medium-sized ripe avocado
a large handful of fresh spinach leaves
60g Greek yoghurt (use dairy free if preferred)
25g vanilla flavour whey or rice protein powder (optional)

for the toppings:
50g fresh blueberries
5g dried banana chips (optional)
1 tsp cocoa nibs
1 tsp chia seeds

SERVES 1

Place the smoothie bowl ingredients in a blender jug and blend well until smooth.

Transfer to a serving bowl.

Add the toppings and serve.

Store any leftovers in an airtight container and refrigerate for up to 2 days.

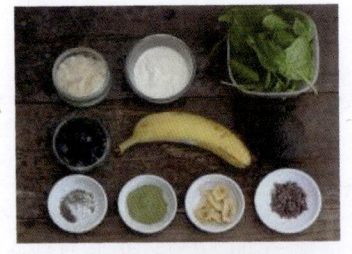

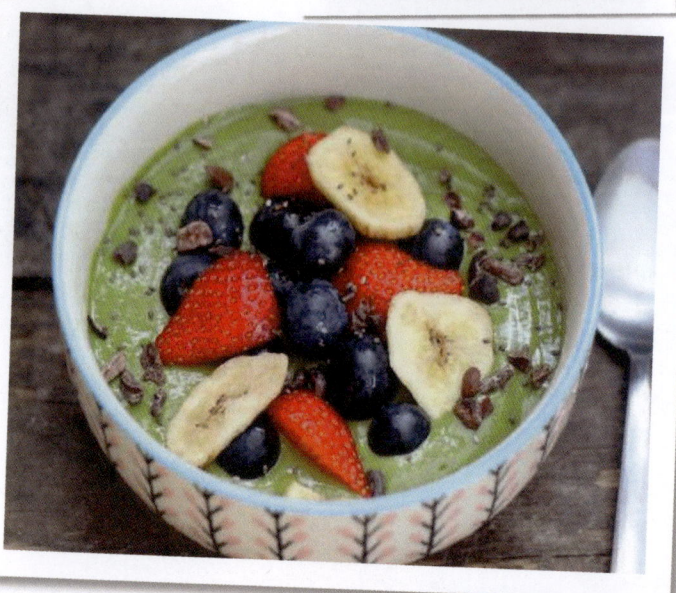

PER SERVING:
429 Calories
40g Carbs
29g Protein
17g Fat

Chickpea breakfast hash

1 tsp coconut oil
½ a small white onion, finely sliced
1 red bell-pepper, diced
150g tinned chickpeas (drained weight), rinsed
1 tsp cumin seeds
½ tsp sea salt
½ tsp ground black pepper
2 eggs
1 tbsp fresh parsley, finely chopped
1 tbsp fresh coriander, finely chopped
25g Feta cheese, crumbled
juice of ½ a lemon

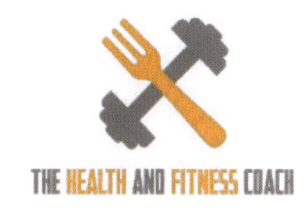

SERVES 1

Heat the oil in a frying pan over a medium heat. Add the onion and bell-pepper and fry for 8-10 minutes, stirring occasionally, until the onion starts to caramelise.

Add the chickpeas, cumin seeds, salt and pepper and stir well.

Using a wooden spoon make two wells in the mixture. Crack an egg into each well and fry for 3 minutes, or until the egg is cooked to your liking.

Sprinkle the parsley, coriander and Feta cheese over the hash.

Transfer to a plate, drizzle the lemon juice over the top and serve.

Consume immediately.

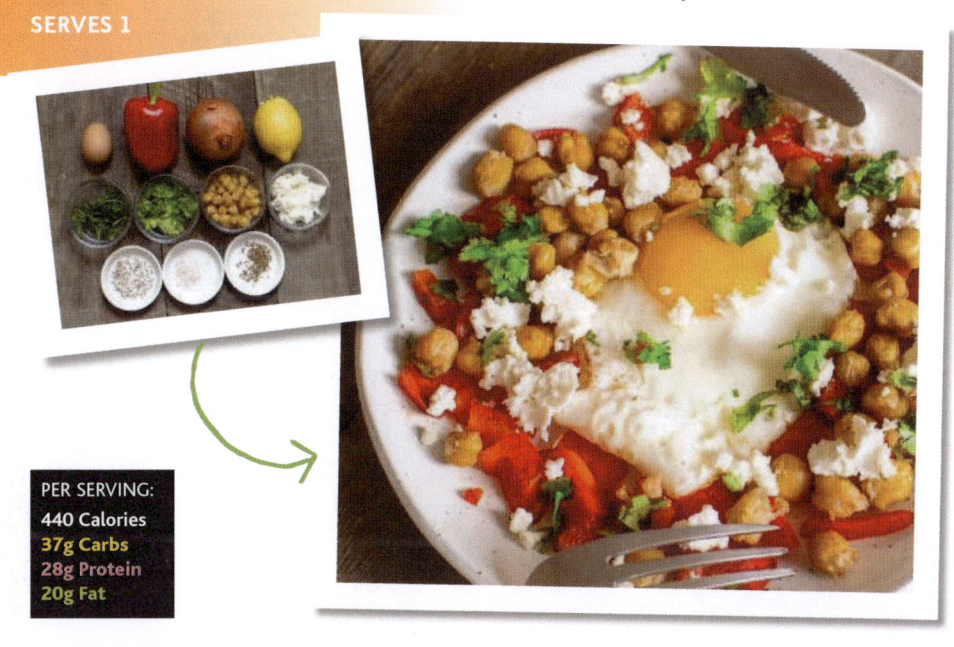

PER SERVING:
440 Calories
37g Carbs
28g Protein
20g Fat

https://thehealthandfitnesscoach.co.uk

BREAKFAST

Mexican scrambled eggs

3 eggs
½ tsp ground cumin
½ tsp sea salt
a pinch of cayenne pepper
20ml whole milk or unsweetened almond milk
½ tbsp butter
30g white onion, diced
30g red bell-pepper, finely sliced
3 jalapeño peppers, finely chopped (optional)

SERVES 1

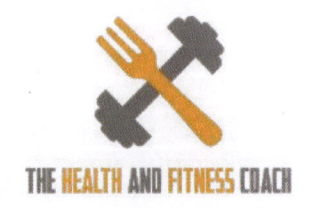

In a bowl, whisk together the eggs, cumin, salt, cayenne pepper and milk.

Heat a skillet over a medium/high heat. Add the butter and heat until melted.

Add the onion and bell-pepper and fry gently for 3-4 minutes, stirring occasionally until soft.

Pour in the egg mixture and allow to cook for 30 seconds, then stir gently, breaking the eggs apart.

Cook for 1-2 minutes, stirring continuously until the eggs are cooked.

Transfer the eggs to a plate. Sprinkle the jalapeños over the eggs and serve.

Consume immediately.

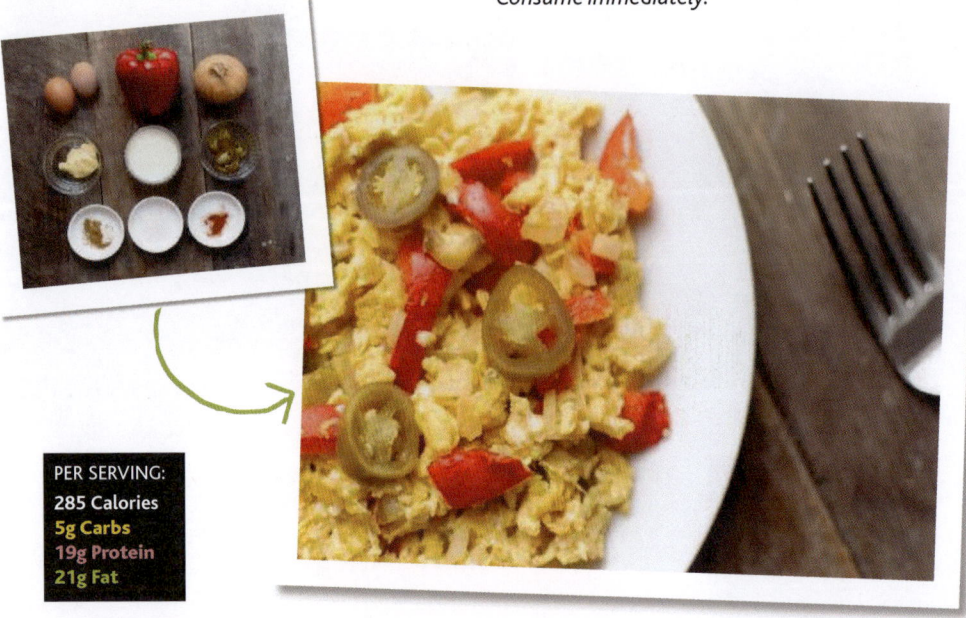

PER SERVING:
285 Calories
5g Carbs
19g Protein
21g Fat

BREAKFAST

Mango overnight oats

100g oats (use gluten free if preferred)
120ml unsweetened almond milk
25g vanilla flavour whey or rice protein powder (optional)
70g Greek yoghurt (use dairy free if preferred)
1 tbsp honey or maple syrup
1 tsp almond or vanilla extract
1 tbsp chia seeds
100g frozen mango chunks

SERVES 2

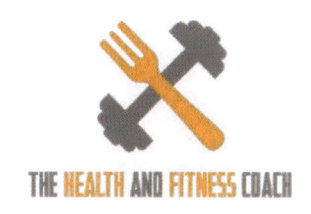

Method 1: Divide the oats between two mason jars. Add the milk, protein powder (if using) and yoghurt. Stir well.

Add the honey and almond extract. Top with the chia seeds and mango.

Refrigerate overnight. Serve.

Method 2: Place all of the ingredients into a sealable container, except for the mango. Stir well.

Refrigerate overnight.

Stir again and add more milk if the mixture is too thick. Transfer to two serving bowls. Top with the mango and serve.

Store any leftovers in an airtight container and refrigerate for up to 2 days.

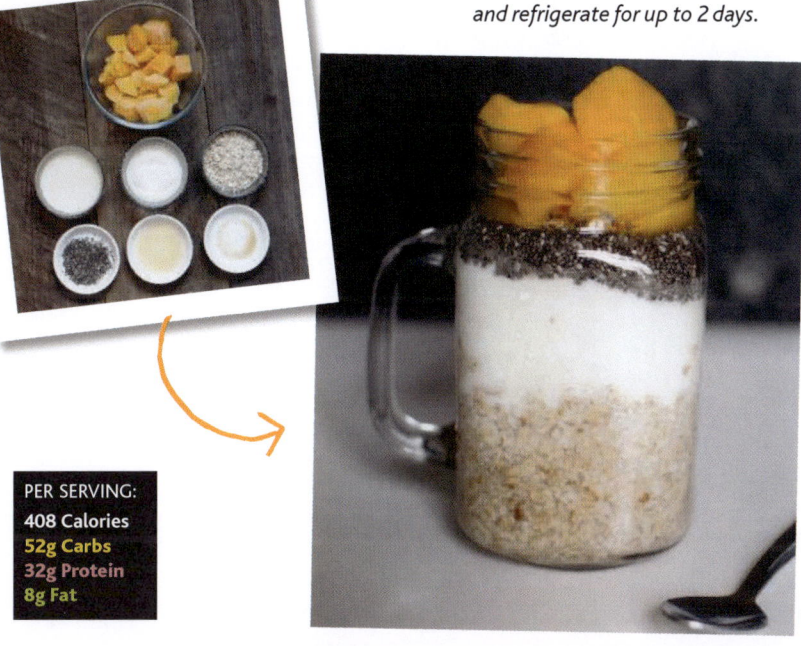

PER SERVING:
408 Calories
52g Carbs
32g Protein
8g Fat

THE HEALTH AND FITNESS COACH

https://thehealthandfitnesscoach.co.uk

BREAKFAST 38

Strawberry cream porridge

60g oats (use gluten free if preferred)
140ml unsweetened almond milk (or use milk of your choice)
90g strawberries
25g strawberry or vanilla flavour whey or rice protein powder
1 tsp chia seeds
1 tsp flaked almonds

SERVES 1

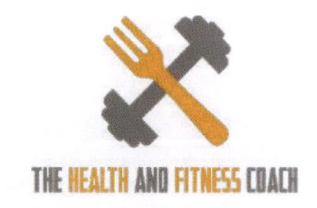

Place the oats and milk in a saucepan over a medium heat. Cook for 2 minutes, stirring. Add more milk if the mixture is too thick.

Add the strawberries and cook for 3-4 minutes, stirring frequently. Add more milk if required.

When the oats are thick and creamy, remove the saucepan from the heat.

Add the protein powder and chia seeds and stir well.

Transfer to a serving bowl and top with the almonds.

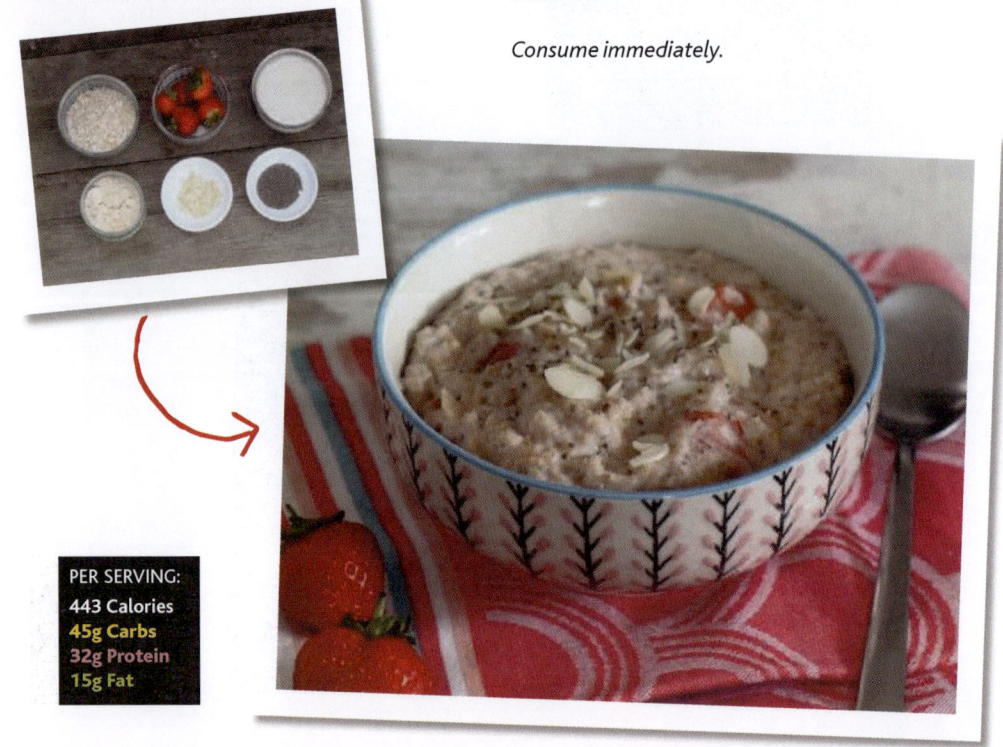

Consume immediately.

PER SERVING:
443 Calories
45g Carbs
32g Protein
15g Fat

https://thehealthandfitnesscoach.co.uk   BREAKFAST   39

Egg breakfast bowl

2 tsps coconut oil
130g cauliflower, roughly chopped
½ tsp ground turmeric
½ tsp medium curry powder
a pinch of sea salt and ground black pepper
40g red onion, sliced
50g fresh spinach
2 eggs
40g ripe avocado, sliced

SERVES 1

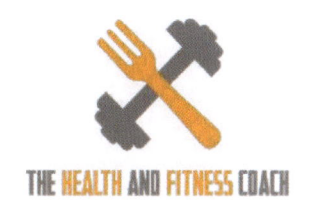

Melt half of the oil in a frying pan over a medium heat. Add the cauliflower, turmeric, curry powder, salt and pepper. Fry gently for 3-4 minutes, stirring frequently.

Add the onion and sauté for 3-4 minutes, stirring frequently.

Add the spinach and cook, stirring frequently, until the spinach has wilted.

Transfer the contents of the pan to a serving bowl.

Add the remaining oil to the frying pan. Crack the eggs carefully into the pan. Fry until the yolks are cooked to your liking.

Transfer the cooked eggs to the serving bowl. Top with sliced avocado. Serve.

Consume immediately.

PER SERVING:
365 Calories
17g Carbs
18g Protein
25g Fat

https://thehealthandfitnesscoach.co.uk

BREAKFAST 40

Quick crunchy muesli

50g oats (use gluten free if preferred)
25g vanilla or strawberry flavour whey or rice protein powder (optional)
130ml unsweetened almond milk (or use milk of your choice)
10g brazil nuts or cashews, roughly chopped
10g almonds or hazelnuts, roughly chopped
10g raisins or sultanas

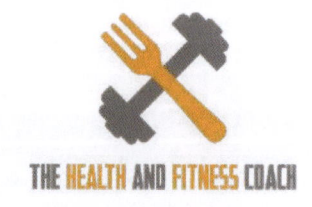

Mix the oats, protein powder (if using) and milk in a bowl.

Allow to stand for 10 minutes. Leave to stand for longer if a thicker consistency is desired. Add a splash more milk if the mixture becomes too thick.

Stir in the remaining ingredients and serve.

Store any leftovers in an airtight container and refrigerate for up to 2 days.

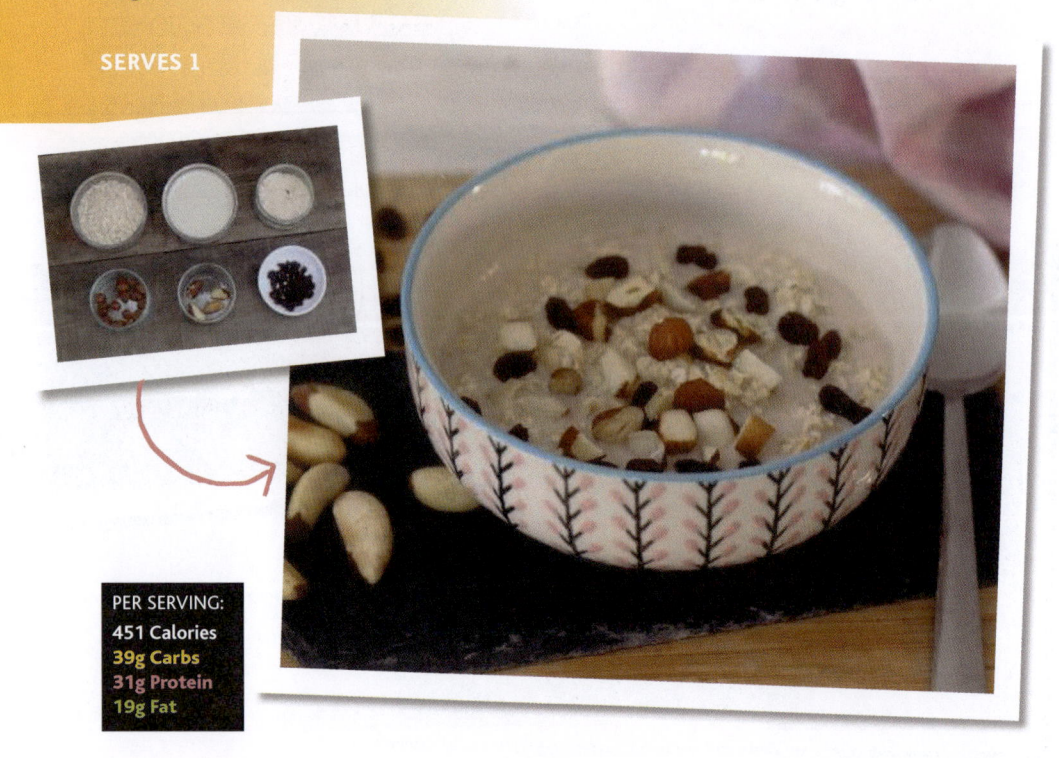

SERVES 1

PER SERVING:
451 Calories
39g Carbs
31g Protein
19g Fat

https://thehealthandfitnesscoach.co.uk

BREAKFAST 41

Oatless nut porridge

10g flaxseed
15g walnuts and / or pecans
5g unsweetened coconut flakes or desiccated coconut
½ tsp ground cinnamon
1 egg
2 egg whites
60ml unsweetened almond milk (or use milk of your choice)
10g cashew or almond butter
60g ripe banana, mashed
½ tsp chia seeds
for the topping:
25g fresh berries of your choice

SERVES 1

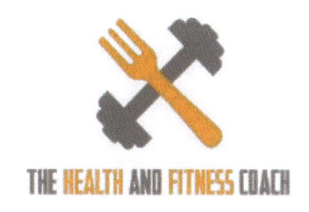

Place the flaxseed, nuts, coconut flakes and cinnamon in a blender or food processor. Blend well until coarsely ground.

Place the egg, egg whites, milk, nut butter and banana in a bowl and blend well using an electric hand blender.

Add the ground nut mixture and chia seeds and stir well until combined.

Transfer the mixture to a saucepan and cook over a medium/low heat, stirring continuously until thick and creamy. Add more milk during cooking time, if the mixture becomes too thick.

Serve topped with fresh berries.

Consume immediately.

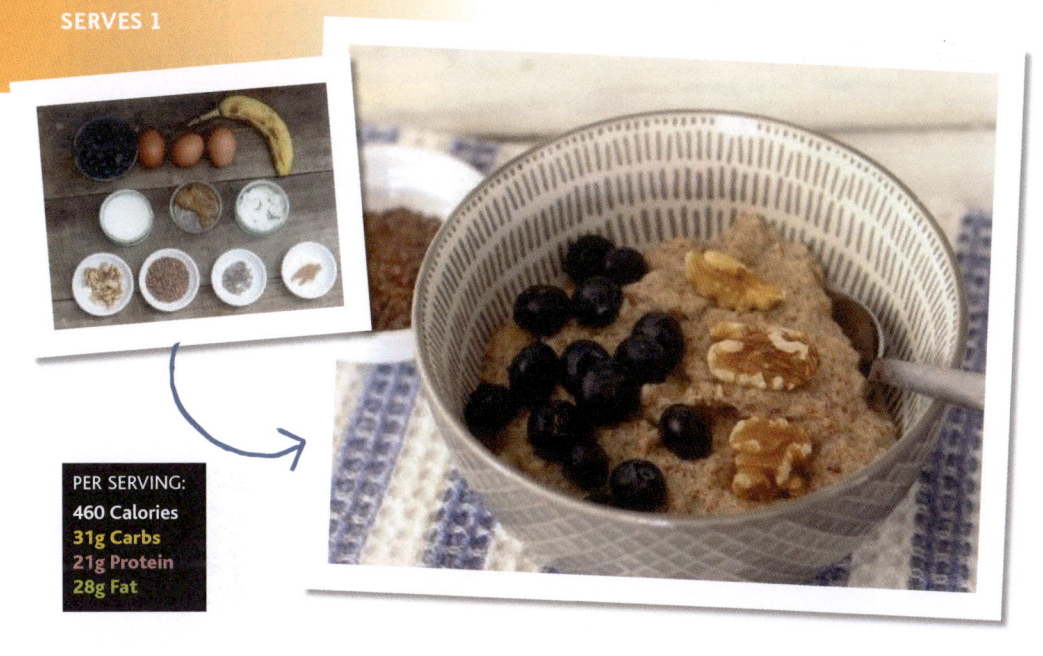

PER SERVING:
460 Calories
31g Carbs
21g Protein
28g Fat

https://thehealthandfitnesscoach.co.uk

BREAKFAST

Creamy baked eggs

1 tsp coconut oil or butter
a small handful kale or spinach leaves, chopped
60g mushrooms (any variety), roughly chopped
1 spring onion, roughly chopped
a pinch of sea salt and ground black pepper
1 garlic clove, finely chopped
a small pinch of dried thyme or mixed herbs
2 tsps crème fraîche
15g Cheddar or Swiss cheese, grated (use dairy free if preferred)
2 eggs

SERVES 1

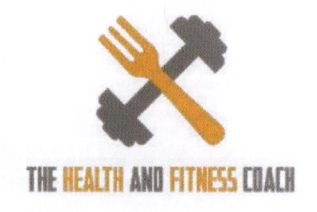

Melt the oil/ butter in a large frying pan over a medium heat.

Add the kale, mushrooms, spring onion, salt and pepper, and stir well. Cook for 4-5 minutes, stirring frequently until softened.

Add the garlic and dried herbs. Cook for 2-3 minutes, stirring continuously.

Add the crème fraîche, stir and remove the pan from the heat. Top with the grated cheese.

Using a spoon, make two wells in the mixture. Carefully crack an egg into each well.

Cover with a lid and cook over a low heat for 4-5 minutes, or until the eggs are cooked to your liking. Serve.

Consume immediately.

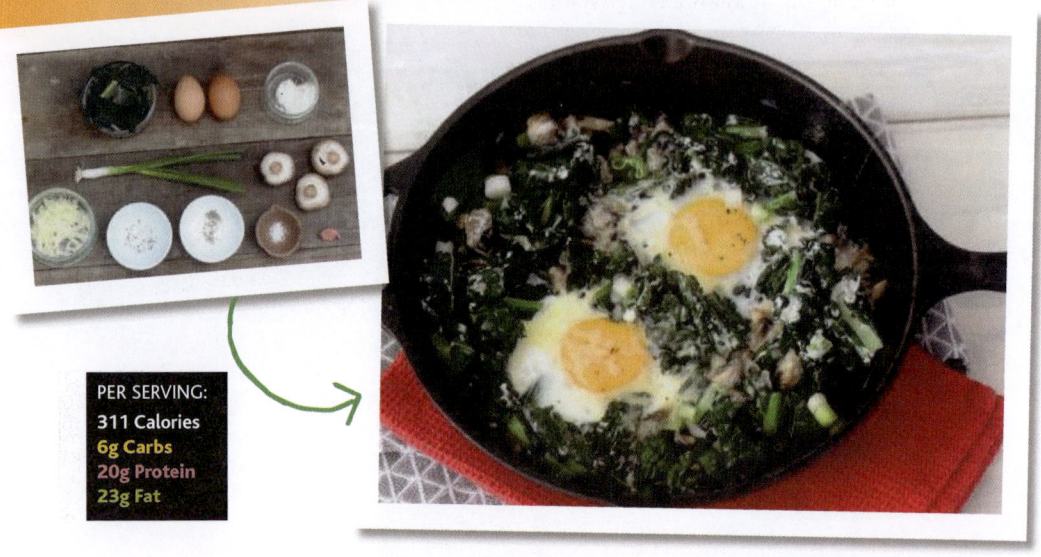

PER SERVING:
311 Calories
6g Carbs
20g Protein
23g Fat

THE HEALTH AND FITNESS COACH

https://thehealthandfitnesscoach.co.uk

BREAKFAST

Feta & spinach breakfast hash

2 eggs
1 egg white
a pinch of sea salt and ground black pepper
¼ tsp paprika
1 tsp coconut oil
60g cherry tomatoes, halved
50g button mushrooms, chopped
50g red bell-pepper, chopped
2 spring onions, chopped
60g fresh spinach leaves
20g Feta cheese, cut into small cubes

SERVES 1

Crack the eggs and egg white into a jug. Add the salt, pepper and paprika and beat with a fork.

Heat the oil in a frying pan over a medium heat. Add the tomatoes, mushrooms, bell-pepper and spring onions and cook for 3-4 minutes, stirring occasionally until soft.

Add the spinach and cook for 2 minutes, stirring occasionally until wilted.

Add the Feta and cook for 1-2 minutes, to heat through.

Pour in the eggs. Stir continuously until thoroughly cooked. Serve.

Consume immediately.

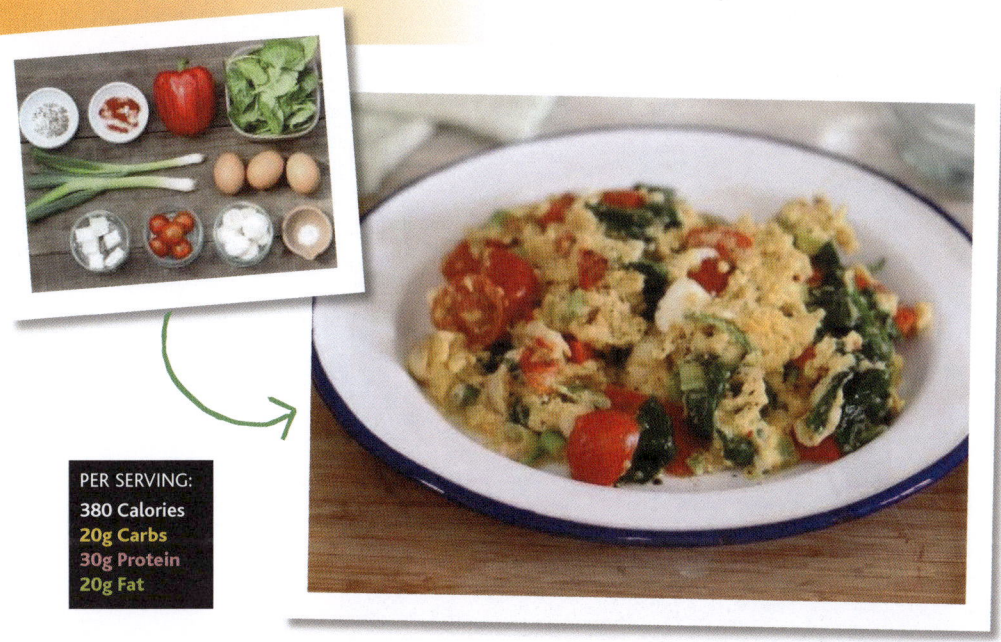

PER SERVING:
380 Calories
20g Carbs
30g Protein
20g Fat

https://thehealthandfitnesscoach.co.uk

BREAKFAST   44

Fluffy berry omelette

3 eggs
15ml unsweetened almond milk or whole milk
¼ tsp ground ginger
½ tsp cinnamon
½ tsp coconut oil
50g cottage cheese or cream cheese
90g fresh berries of your choice, chopped
juice of ½ a lemon
to serve:
a few fresh mint leaves (optional)
a few extra berries

SERVES 1

Crack the eggs into a jug. Add the milk, ginger and cinnamon and beat gently with a fork.

Heat the oil in a large frying pan or skillet and pour in the egg mixture. Tilt the pan gently to cover the base. Cook for 2-3 minutes, or until the omelette has set. Transfer to a plate.

Top with the cheese, berries and lemon juice. Fold in half and cut into quarters.

Serve garnished with mint leaves, if using, and a few extra berries.

Consume immediately.

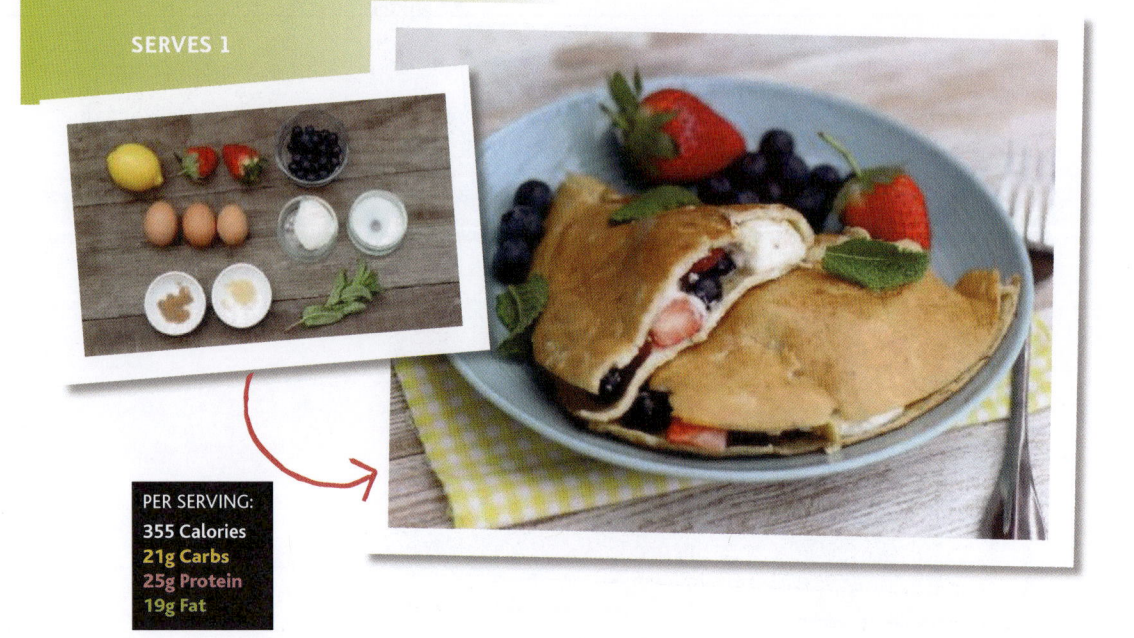

PER SERVING:
355 Calories
21g Carbs
25g Protein
19g Fat

https://thehealthandfitnesscoach.co.uk

BREAKFAST 45

Kale, bacon & egg fry up

½ tsp coconut oil
3 unsmoked bacon rashers, visible fat removed and chopped
60g white onion, diced
60g closed-cup mushrooms, sliced
½ a green or red bell-pepper, diced
40g kale, chopped
½ tsp garlic granules
a small pinch of red chilli flakes
a pinch of sea salt
4 eggs

SERVES 2

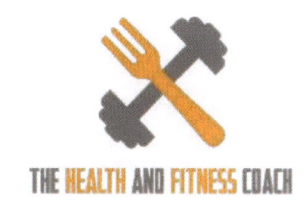

Preheat oven to 200°C/400°F.

Melt the oil in a skillet or ovenproof frying pan over a medium heat. Add the bacon and cook until crispy on both sides. Transfer to a plate lined with kitchen roll.

Reduce the heat to medium/low. Add the onion, mushrooms and bell-pepper to the frying pan and fry for 3-4 minutes, or until soft.

Add the kale, garlic granules, chilli flakes and salt. Stir well, cover and cook for 2-3 minutes, or until the kale is soft. Remove the pan from the heat and stir in the cooked bacon.

Make 4 small wells in the kale for the eggs to sit. Crack an egg carefully into each well. Bake for 5-6 minutes depending on how you like your eggs cooked. Serve.

Consume immediately.

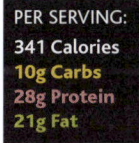

PER SERVING:
341 Calories
10g Carbs
28g Protein
21g Fat

THE HEALTH AND FITNESS COACH

https://thehealthandfitnesscoach.co.uk

BREAKFAST 46

Scrambled eggs with a twist

THE HEALTH AND FITNESS COACH

2 eggs
3 egg whites
½ tsp chilli flakes
¾ tsp mustard (any variety)
a pinch of sea salt and ground black pepper
1 tsp coconut oil or butter

SERVES 1

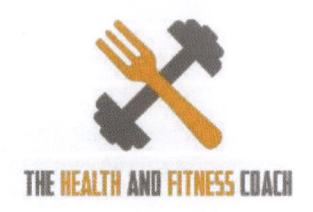

Crack the eggs and egg whites into a jug. Add the chilli flakes, mustard, salt and pepper.

Melt the oil / butter in a frying pan over a medium heat.

Add the egg mixture and cook gently, stirring continuously until the eggs are cooked through. Serve.

Consume immediately.

Serving suggestion:

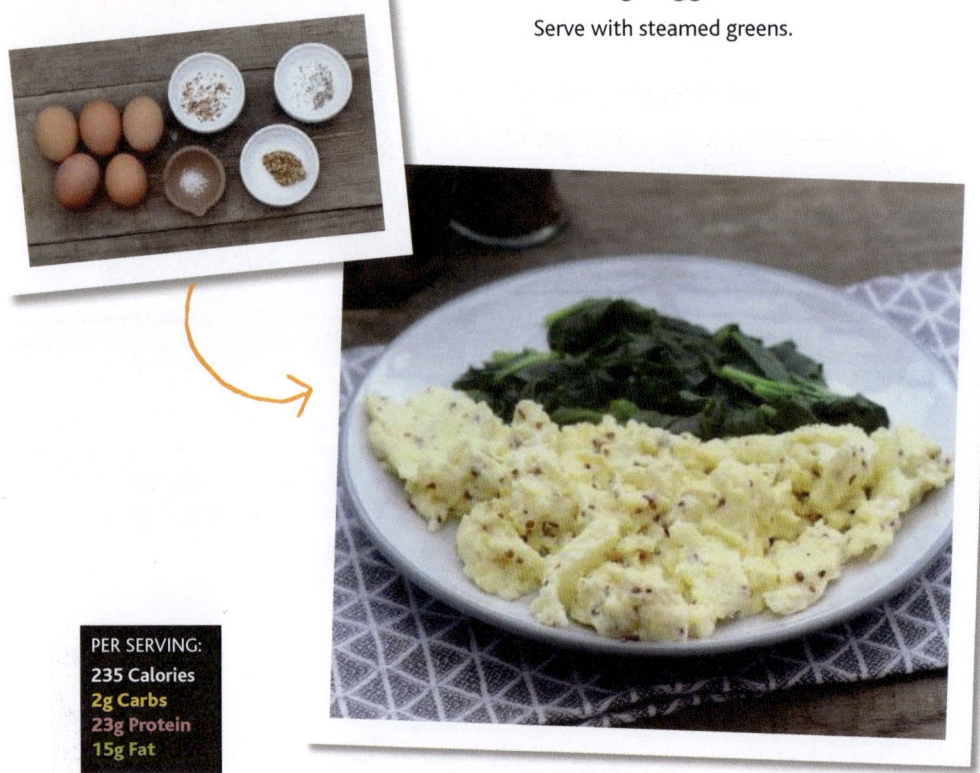

Serve with steamed greens.

PER SERVING:
235 Calories
2g Carbs
23g Protein
15g Fat

https://thehealthandfitnesscoach.co.uk

BREAKFAST 47

Quinoa veggie bake

25g quinoa (uncooked weight)
1 tsp coconut oil, to grease dish
3 egg whites
2 eggs
a pinch of sea salt and ground black pepper
½ a red bell-pepper, diced
60g closed-cup or button mushrooms, chopped
60g red onion, finely chopped
½ a medium-sized ripe avocado, diced
½ tsp paprika
¼ tsp hot chilli powder
¼ tsp garlic granules
30g Cheddar cheese, grated (use dairy free if preferred)

MAKES 9 SLICES

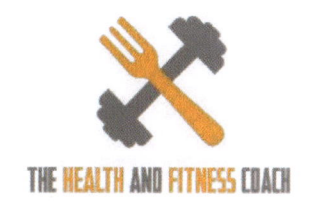

Rinse the quinoa in cold water. Bring a small saucepan of water to the boil. Add the quinoa and cook according to packet instructions. Transfer to a sieve, rinse in cold water to cool, then drain well. Pat dry with kitchen roll to remove excess moisture.

Preheat oven to 180°C/350°F.

Grease the base and sides of a 15x15cm ovenproof dish or baking tin with coconut oil.

Crack the eggs and whites into a jug. Add the salt and pepper and beat gently with a fork. Add the remaining ingredients and stir well. Transfer the mixture to the ovenproof dish. Bake for 25-30 minutes, or until firm.

Cut into 9 slices and remove from the tin using a fish slice. Serve warm or cold.

Store any leftovers in an airtight container and refrigerate for up to 2 days.

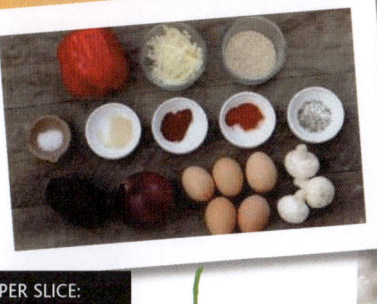

PER SLICE:
68 Calories
4g Carbs
4g Protein
4g Fat

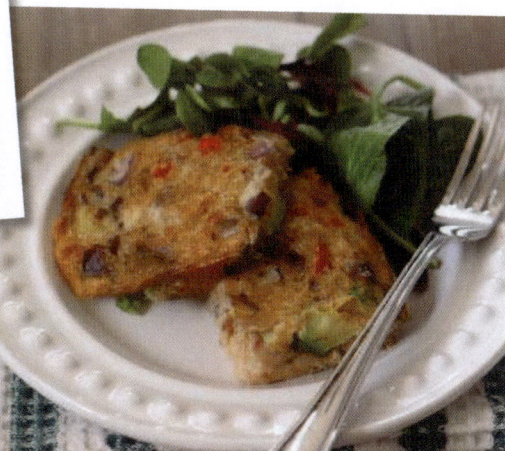

THE HEALTH AND FITNESS COACH

https://thehealthandfitnesscoach.co.uk

BREAKFAST 48

Chicken fattoush

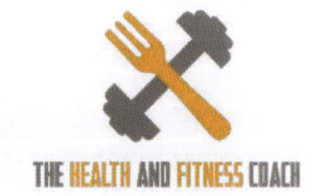

2 vine-ripened tomatoes, chopped
80g cucumber, sliced
60g red onion, sliced
1 small lettuce (any variety), shredded
a handful of fresh mint leaves, roughly chopped
a handful of fresh parsley leaves, finely chopped
1 tsp sumac (or substitute with 1 tsp finely grated lemon zest)

for the shredded chicken:
2 x 150g chicken breasts
1 tsp black pepper
½ - 1 tsp sea salt

for the dressing:
½ a garlic clove, peeled and crushed
2 tbsps malt vinegar
1 tbsp extra virgin olive oil
juice of ½ a lemon
1 tsp sumac (or substitute with 1 tsp finely grated lemon zest)

SERVES 2

Place the chicken breast into a large saucepan. Season with salt and pepper. Cover with 1 inch of cold water.

Place the saucepan over a medium/high heat and bring the water to a boil. Reduce heat and simmer for 10 minutes, or until the chicken has cooked throughout.

Remove the chicken from the water and transfer to a plate to cool. Shred with a fork.

Arrange the salad ingredients in two serving bowls. Top with the chicken.

Mix the dressing ingredients in a jug and drizzle over the salads. Serve.

Store any leftovers in an airtight container and refrigerate for up to 2 days.

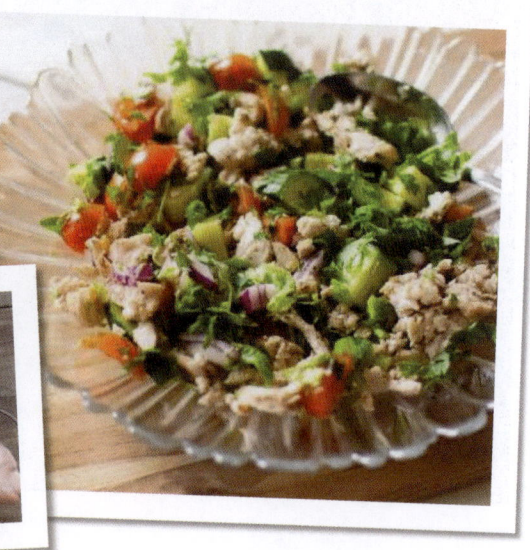

PER SERVING:
269 Calories
14g Carbs
33g Protein
9g Fat

Lemon & herb chicken

10 chicken legs, skin removed
juice of ½ a lemon
1 lemon, sliced
60ml olive oil
2 garlic cloves, minced
2 tsps sea salt
½ tsp ground black pepper
1 tsp paprika
1 tsp dried oregano
1 tsp cayenne pepper
1 tsp fresh or dried thyme
1 tsp garlic powder (optional)

SERVES 5

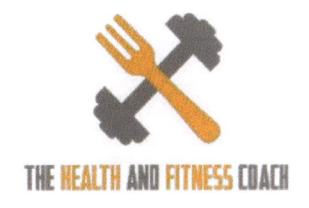

Pat the chicken dry using kitchen roll. Place in a large bowl.

Mix the remaining ingredients in a jug (except for the lemon slices). Pour over the chicken.

Cover and refrigerate for 2 hours, or overnight if you have time.

Remove the chicken from the fridge and allow to rest at room temperature for 20 minutes.

Preheat oven to 180°C/350°F.

Place the chicken onto a foil-lined baking tray. Arrange the lemon slices over the chicken legs. Bake for 20-25 minutes. Turn the chicken over and cook for 10 minutes or until thoroughly cooked. When cooked, the juices will run clear when pierced with a skewer.

Store any leftovers in an airtight container and refrigerate for up to 3 days.

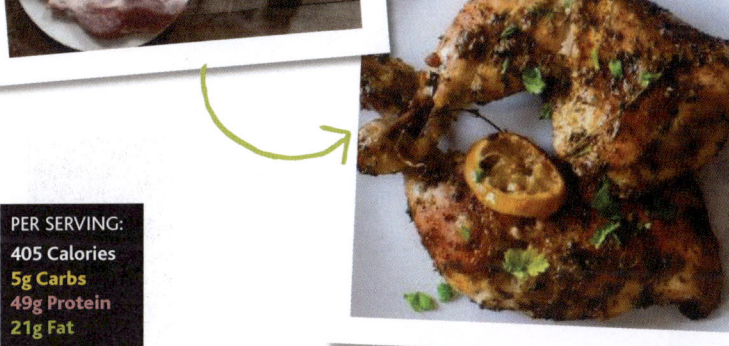

PER SERVING:
405 Calories
5g Carbs
49g Protein
21g Fat

https://thehealthandfitnesscoach.co.uk

LUNCH

Courgetti carbonara

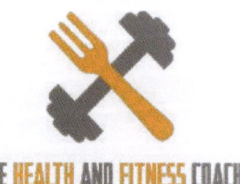

2 egg yolks
2 tbsps crème fraîche or plain yoghurt (use dairy free if preferred)
a pinch of sea salt and ground black pepper
2 tbsps parmesan, finely grated (use dairy free if preferred)
1 tsp coconut oil
1 garlic clove, crushed or finely chopped
100g cooked ham, chopped (optional)
400g courgettes, spiralised (or cut into ribbons with a potato peeler
a sprinkle of fresh parsley, finely chopped

SERVES 2

Whisk the egg yolks, crème fraîche, salt, pepper and parmesan in a bowl.

Heat the coconut oil in a frying pan over a medium heat. Add the garlic and cook for one minute.

Add the courgettes to the frying pan, stir well and cook for one minute. Add the ham and cook for one more minute.

Remove from the heat, add in the cream mixture and stir well to coat the courgette. Stir continuously, until the sauce is warmed through.

Serve garnished with fresh chopped parsley.

Consume immediately.

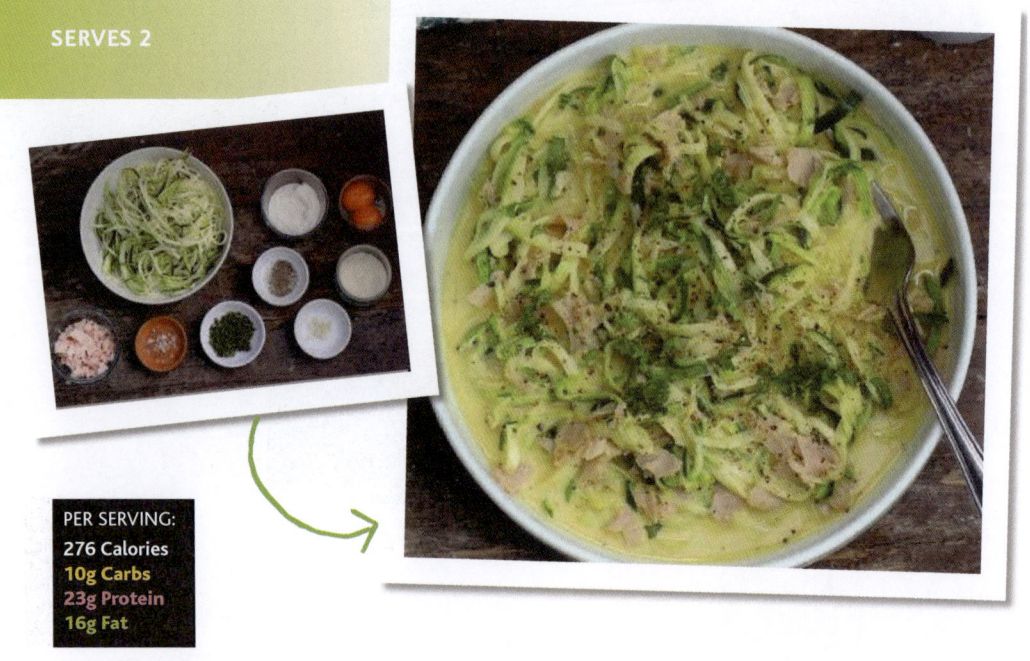

PER SERVING:
276 Calories
10g Carbs
23g Protein
16g Fat

https://thehealthandfitnesscoach.co.uk

LUNCH 51

Crustless tomato & basil quiche

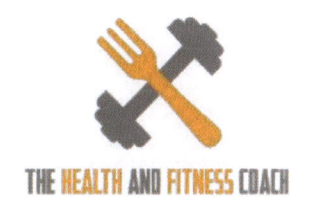

a small amount of coconut oil or butter, to grease dish
2 vine-ripened tomatoes
4 eggs
2 egg whites
¼ tsp Italian herbs
½ tsp paprika
a pinch of sea salt and ground black pepper
4 spring onions, finely sliced
100g plain cottage cheese
35g Swiss cheese, finely grated
20g Parmesan cheese, finely grated
10 basil leaves, chopped

SERVES 3

Preheat oven to 180°C/350°F. Lightly grease a medium-sized oven dish with coconut oil or butter.

Finely slice one of the tomatoes and finely chop the other.

Crack the eggs and whites into a jug. Add the Italian herbs, paprika, salt and pepper and stir well.

Stir in the chopped tomato, spring onions, and cheese. Pour the mixture into the dish. Bake for 40 minutes.

Distribute the tomato slices evenly around the surface of the quiche. Add the chopped basil. Bake for 20 minutes, or until the centre of the quiche is cooked.

Cut into 3 pieces. Serve warm or cold.

Store any leftovers in an airtight container and refrigerate for up to 2 days.

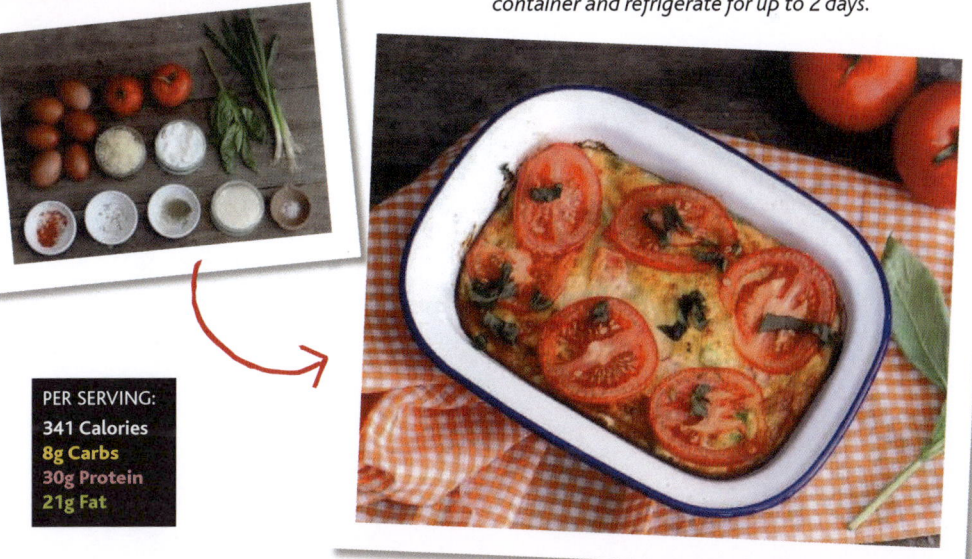

PER SERVING:
341 Calories
8g Carbs
30g Protein
21g Fat

https://thehealthandfitnesscoach.co.uk

LUNCH

Smokey chicken & mixed bean soup

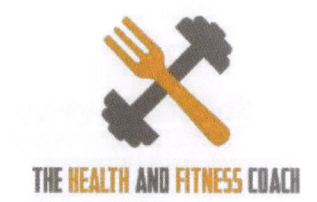

1 tsp ghee or coconut oil
1 medium-sized white onion, chopped
1 red bell-pepper, diced
1 yellow bell-pepper, diced
2 garlic cloves, finely chopped
400g tinned tomatoes
250ml cold water
250g fresh chicken breast strips
400g tinned mixed beans, drained
150ml tinned coconut milk

for the spice mix:
a pinch of sea salt and black pepper
1 tsp ground cumin
1 tsp chipotle flakes
2 tsps smoked paprika
1 tsp chilli flakes

to serve:
¼ a medium-sized avocado (per person), sliced
a small bunch of fresh coriander, finely chopped

SERVES 3

Heat the ghee/oil in a large saucepan over a medium heat. Add the onion and sauté for 4 minutes, stirring occasionally.

Add the bell-peppers and garlic and fry for 3 minutes, stirring occasionally.

Add the spice mix, tinned tomatoes and cold water. Stir well, increase heat and bring to a boil. Reduce heat and simmer gently for 10 minutes. Taste and add more seasoning if required.

Add the chicken, stir well and cook for 10 minutes. Add the mixed beans, stir well and cook for 5 minutes. Add the coconut milk, stir well and cook for 1 minute.

Serve topped with avocado and coriander.

Store any leftovers in an airtight container and refrigerate for up to 3 days or freeze on same day.

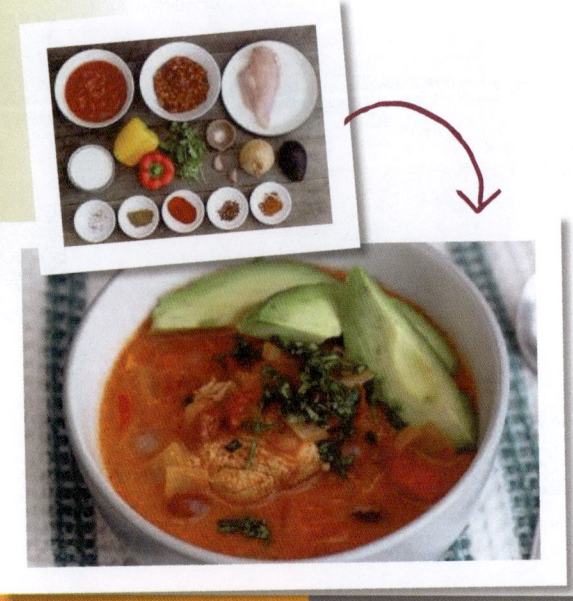

PER SERVING:
402 Calories
38g Carbs
31g Protein
14g Fat

THE HEALTH AND FITNESS COACH

https://thehealthandfitnesscoach.co.uk

LUNCH

Blackened salmon with roasted vegetables

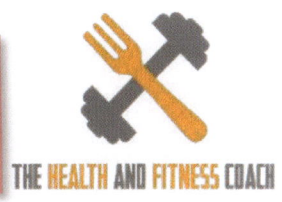

1 heaped tsp coconut oil, melted
2 x 150g fresh salmon fillets
1 small red onion, sliced
2 vine ripened tomatoes, cut into segments
120g Tenderstem broccoli
a large handful of kale
a sprinkle of sunflower seeds

for the seasoning:
1 heaped tsp ground cumin
½ tsp smoked paprika
½ tsp ground fennel seeds
½ tsp cayenne pepper
½ tsp garlic powder
½ tsp sea salt
½ tsp ground black pepper

SERVES 2

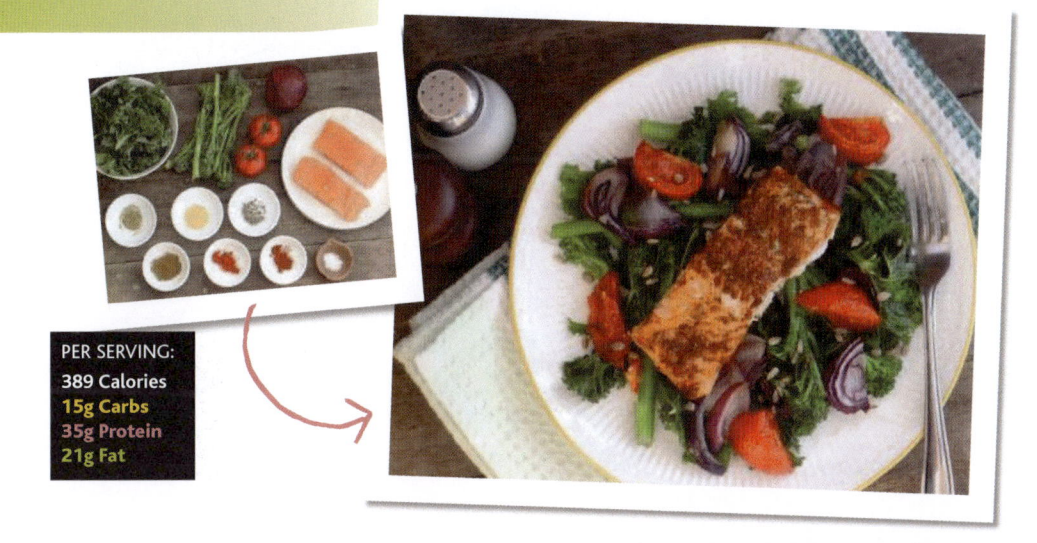

Preheat oven to 180°C/350°F.

Mix the seasoning in a small bowl. Add the melted coconut oil and stir well.

Spoon the seasoning mixture over the salmon fillets, and spread evenly to cover the tops.

Place the salmon on a large foil lined oven tray. Add the tomatoes and onion, and spread to distribute evenly.

Bake for 25 minutes, or until the salmon is cooked and the onion is soft.

Steam the broccoli and kale for 3-4 minutes, or until tender. Serve topped with the sunflower seeds.

Store any leftover salmon fillets in an airtight container and refrigerate for up to 2 days.

PER SERVING:
389 Calories
15g Carbs
35g Protein
21g Fat

Carrot & coriander soup

2 tsps ghee or coconut oil
1 medium-sized white onion, finely chopped
1 garlic clove, minced
1 large white potato, peeled and chopped
450g carrots, peeled and chopped
1.1l vegetable stock (made with one organic stock cube)
1 tsp ground coriander
a pinch of sea salt and ground black pepper
a handful of fresh handful coriander, chopped

SERVES 3

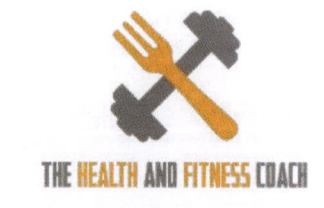

Heat the ghee/oil in a large saucepan. Add the onion and garlic and fry for 6 minutes, or until softened.

Add the potato and carrots and fry for 3-4 minutes, stirring occasionally.

Add the stock, ground coriander, salt and pepper and bring to a boil, then reduce the heat to simmer.

Cover and cook for 20-25 minutes, or until the carrots are tender.

Pour into a food processor add most of the fresh coriander and blitz well to desired consistency.

Serve garnished with the remaining fresh coriander.

Store any leftovers in an airtight container and refrigerate for up to 3 days or freeze on same day.

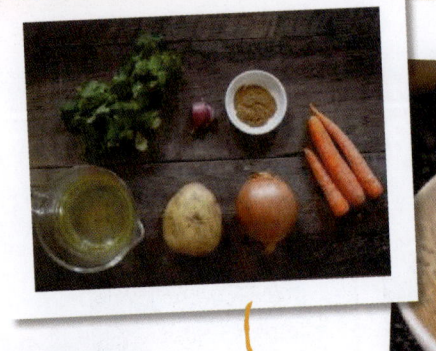

PER SERVING:
200 Calories
37g Carbs
4g Protein
4g Fat

https://thehealthandfitnesscoach.co.uk

LUNCH

Vegan chickpea wraps

for the flatbread:
120g plain flour (use gluten free flour if preferred)
1 tsp baking powder
½ tsp sea salt
200ml water
a small amount of butter, to grease pan

for the chickpeas:
250g tinned chickpeas (drained weight)
½ tbsp extra virgin olive oil
½ garlic clove, minced
½ tsp sea salt
½ tsp ground cumin
a small pinch of black pepper

for the filling:
1 vine-ripened tomato, sliced
100g ripe avocado, sliced
¼ small red onion, sliced
30g spinach or lettuce leaves

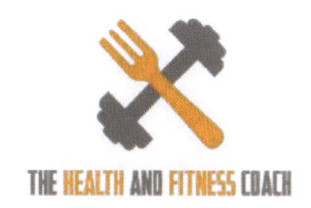

SERVES 2

Drain and rinse the chickpeas and pat dry with kitchen roll.

Place the chickpea ingredients in a food processor (or use an immersion hand blender). Blend well until to form a crumb-like consistency. Taste and add more seasoning if required.

Place the flatbread ingredients in a bowl. Mix well until smooth.

Lightly grease a large frying pan with melted butter. Pour half of the flour mixture into the frying pan and cook for 2-3 minutes, or until bubbles appear on the surface. Turn over and cook for 2-3 minutes. Transfer to a plate.

Repeat steps with remaining mixture.

Spread the chickpea paste across the centre of each flatbread. Add the remaining fillings. Wrap the flatbreads up and slice in half. Serve.

Store any leftovers in an airtight container and refrigerate for up to 1 day.

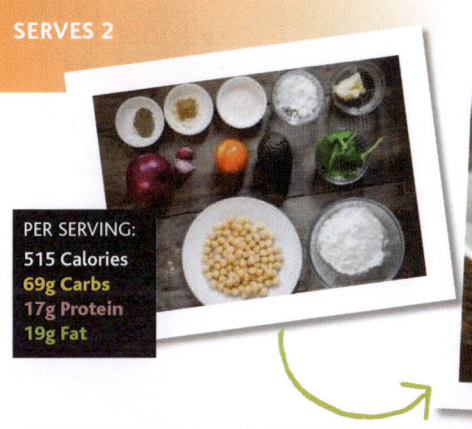

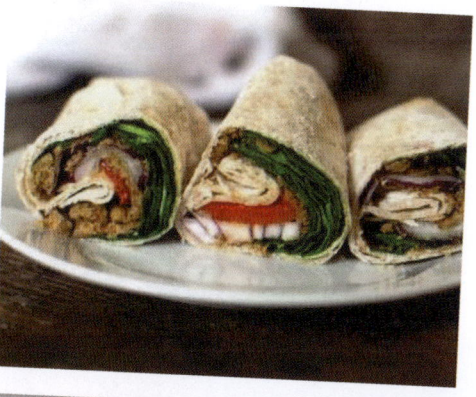

PER SERVING:
515 Calories
69g Carbs
17g Protein
19g Fat

LUNCH

Chipotle chicken & veggie bowl

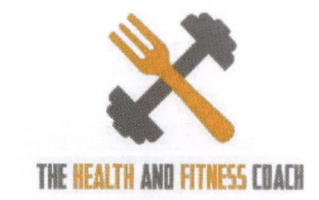

THE HEALTH AND FITNESS COACH

50g uncooked quinoa or amaranth
300g chicken breast, cut into strips
2 tsps chipotle spice blend
1 tsp paprika
a pinch of sea salt and ground black pepper
150g butternut squash, peeled, seeds removed and diced
½ a small red onion, quartered
½ a red bell-pepper, sliced
150g courgette, sliced
1 tbsp olive oil
1 tsp coconut oil
a large handful of rocket leaves
4 cherry tomatoes, halved
20g feta cheese cubes
a drizzle of lemon juice

SERVES 2

Place the quinoa / amaranth in a saucepan of water and cook according to packet instructions. Drain well and set aside.

Preheat oven to 200°C/400°F. Line a baking tray with foil.

Place the spices in a wide-based bowl. Add the chicken and stir well to coat. Cover and refrigerate for 30 minutes.

Spread the squash, onion, bell-pepper and courgette onto the tray. Drizzle over the olive oil. Season with a little salt and pepper, if desired. Roast for 20–25 minutes, or until the vegetables are cooked.

Meanwhile, heat the coconut oil in a frying pan over a medium heat. Add the chicken and cook for around 7-8 minutes, or until thoroughly cooked.

Place the cooked quinoa / amaranth into two serving bowls. Add the remaining ingredients and serve.

Store any leftovers in an airtight container and refrigerate for up to 1 day.

PER SERVING:
494 Calories
42g Carbs
41g Protein
18g Fat

https://thehealthandfitnesscoach.co.uk

LUNCH

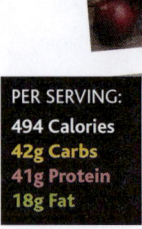

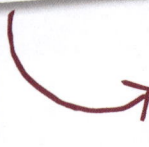

BBQ chicken wings

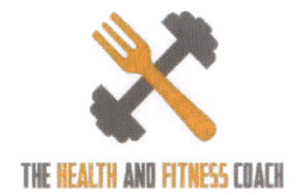

1 tsp sesame seeds
1 spring onion, sliced

for the chicken:
600g chicken wings, skin on
1½ tbsps olive oil
½ tsp sea salt
1 tsp garlic powder
1 tsp smoked paprika
½ tsp ground black pepper

for the BBQ sauce:
1 tsp ghee or coconut oil
1 small white onion, finely chopped
300g tinned chopped tomatoes
2 garlic cloves, finely chopped
2 tbsps honey
2½ tbsps malt vinegar
1½ tbsps Worcestershire sauce
2 tsps tomato purée

SERVES 3

Preheat oven to 220°C/450°F. Line a baking tray with foil.

Place the chicken wings in a large bowl. Add the oil and seasonings and mix well.

Place the chicken onto the baking tray. Bake for 15 minutes, then turn over and bake for another 15 minutes.

Meanwhile, heat the ghee/oil in a saucepan over a low heat. Add the onion and fry for 5 minutes, or until soft.

Add the remaining sauce ingredients and stir. Bring the mixture to a boil, then reduce the heat and simmer for 25 minutes, or until the mixture becomes thicker.

Remove from the heat and allow to cool. Blend the mixture until smooth using a hand blender. Taste and add more honey, if required.

Coat the cooked wings with the sauce. Bake the wings for 10 minutes or until glossy. Serve garnished with spring onion and sesame seeds.

Store any leftovers in an airtight container and refrigerate for up to 3 days.

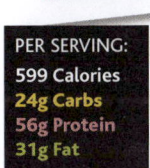

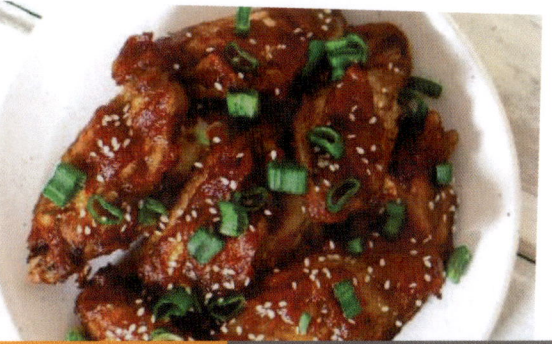

PER SERVING:
599 Calories
24g Carbs
56g Protein
31g Fat

https://thehealthandfitnesscoach.co.uk

LUNCH

Salmon crustless quiche

1 tsp coconut oil, plus extra for greasing
1 small white onion, finely diced
100g fresh spinach or kale
a small pinch of dried mixed herbs
100g mushrooms, cut into ½ cm slices
4 eggs and 1 egg white, beaten
180ml unsweetened almond milk (or use milk of your choice)
a small pinch of sea salt
a small pinch of ground black pepper
50g Cheddar cheese, grated (use dairy free if preferred)
150g smoked salmon

SERVES 2

Preheat oven to 200°C/400°F. Lightly grease the base and sides of an ovenproof dish with coconut oil.

Melt the remaining oil in a large frying pan over a medium heat. Add the onion and sauté for 5 minutes, or until soft and translucent.

Add the spinach, mixed herbs and mushrooms. Cook for 3 minutes, or until the mushrooms have softened slightly. Turn off the heat and allow to cool for 5 minutes.

Put the eggs, milk, salt, black pepper and cheese in a large bowl. Stir well. Add the salmon and cooked vegetables and stir.

Pour into the baking dish. Bake for 35-40 minutes, or until firm in the centre.

Slice in half and serve.

Store any leftovers in an airtight container and refrigerate for up to 2 days or freeze on same day.

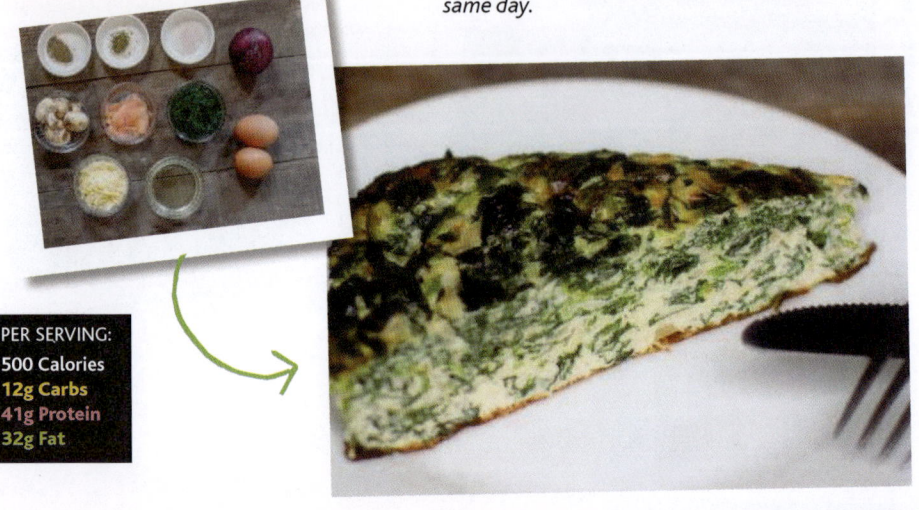

PER SERVING:
500 Calories
12g Carbs
41g Protein
32g Fat

https://thehealthandfitnesscoach.co.uk   LUNCH

Egg salad

4 eggs
1 romaine lettuce head
2 spring onions, finely sliced
¼ tsp paprika
¼ tsp sea salt
¼ tsp ground black pepper
1 tbsp fresh parsley, finely sliced

for the mayonnaise:
1 egg yolk
1 tsp Dijon mustard, at room temperature
1 tsp olive oil
2 tsp white vinegar

SERVES 2

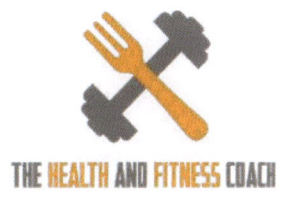

Mix the egg yolk and mustard using an electric hand blender. Slowly add the oil whilst blending. Continue mixing until all of the oil has been combined.

Add the vinegar and mix briefly to combine. Cover and refrigerate. This will allow the mayonnaise to thicken.

Fill a saucepan with water and bring to a boil. Reduce the heat to medium / low. Add the eggs and cook for 10 minutes.

Remove the eggs from the hot water and allow to cool. Peel and chop the eggs, then place into a bowl.

Arrange the lettuce leaves onto a large plate.

Stir the mayonnaise, mustard, spring onion, salt, pepper and paprika into the eggs. Spoon the eggs into the leaves. Garnish with parsley and serve.

Store any leftovers in an airtight container and refrigerate for up to 2 days.

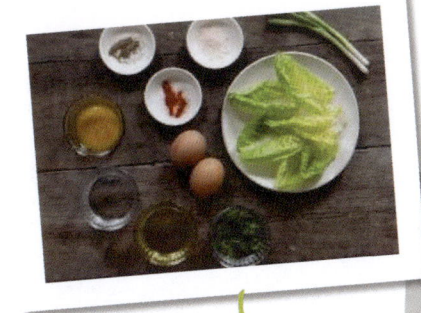

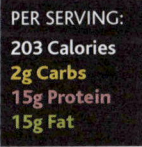

THE HEALTH AND FITNESS COACH

PER SERVING:
203 Calories
2g Carbs
15g Protein
15g Fat

https://thehealthandfitnesscoach.co.uk

LUNCH   60

Red lentil soup

1 tbsp coconut oil
1 medium-sized white onion, peeled and coarsely grated
2 celery stalks, diced
½ tsp sea salt
½ tsp ground black pepper
1 tsp ground cumin
3 garlic cloves, finely chopped
150g red lentils (uncooked), rinsed
1 litre vegetable stock (made with one organic stock cube)
1 ripe salad tomato, diced
3 tsps lemon juice
1 tbsp fresh parsley, finely chopped

SERVES 4

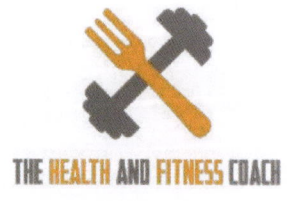

THE HEALTH AND FITNESS COACH

Heat the oil in a large saucepan over a medium heat. Add the onion and celery and sauté for 5 minutes, stirring occasionally.

Add the salt, pepper, cumin and garlic. Stir and fry for one minute.

Add the lentils, stock and tomato. Stir and bring to a boil. Reduce heat and simmer for 20 minutes.

Remove from the heat and add the lemon juice. Taste and add more seasoning if required.

Serve garnished with parsley.

Store any leftovers in an airtight container and refrigerate for up to 3 days or freeze on same day.

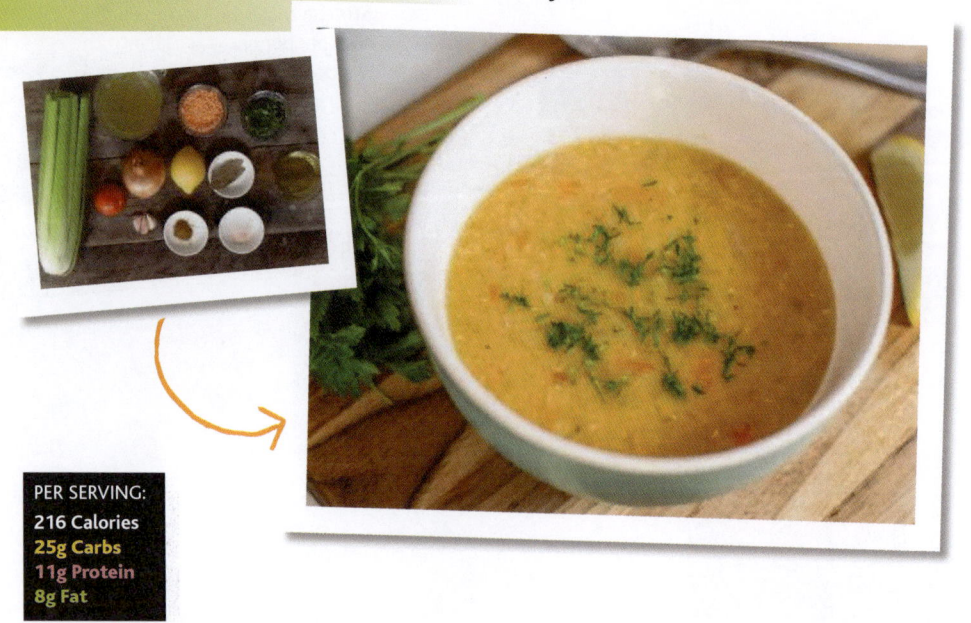

PER SERVING:
216 Calories
25g Carbs
11g Protein
8g Fat

https://thehealthandfitnesscoach.co.uk

Cinnamon chicken

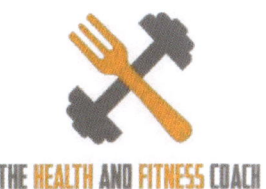

1 tbsp coconut oil
1 medium-sized red onion, diced
2 garlic cloves, finely chopped
2 chicken legs, skin on
½ tbsp allspice or baharat
1 tsp paprika
1 tsp ground cumin
1 tsp sea salt
1 tsp ground black pepper
½ tbsp ground cinnamon
3 tbsps tomato purée
800ml recently boiled water
1 tbsp fresh parsley, chopped

SERVES 2

Heat the oil in a large saucepan over a medium heat. Add the onion and fry gently for 4 minutes, stirring occasionally.

Add the garlic and fry for one minute, stirring occasionally.

Add the chicken legs and brown for 5 minutes, stirring occasionally.

Add the allspice, paprika, cumin, salt, black pepper, cinnamon and tomato purée and stir well. Add the water and bring to a boil.

Cover and simmer for one hour, or until the water has reduced. Stir well and add more water if required during cooking time.

Plate up the chicken either with or without the fried onions in garlic. Serve garnished with parsley.

Store any leftovers in an airtight container and refrigerate for up to 3 days or freeze on same day.

Serving suggestion:

Serve with a mixed salad

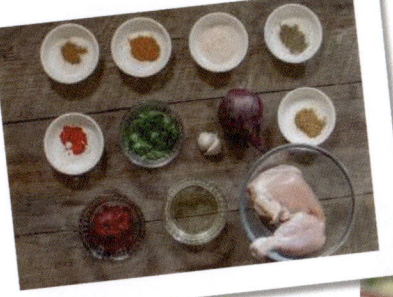

PER SERVING:
366 Calories
14g Carbs
28g Protein
22g Fat

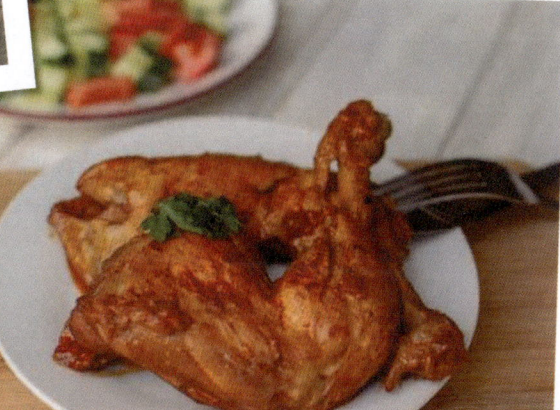

https://thehealthandfitnesscoach.co.uk

LUNCH

Sweet potato frittata

1 tbsp ghee or olive oil
1 medium-sized sweet potato, peeled and diced
1 small white onion, finely diced
6 large eggs
50g Mature Cheddar cheese, grated (use dairy free if preferred)
100ml milk of your choice
1 tsp apple cider vinegar
a small handful of curly kale, roughly chopped
1 tbsp Dijon mustard

SERVES 4

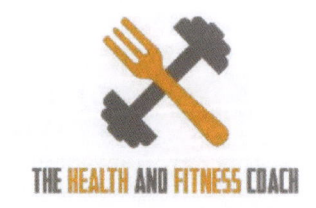

Preheat oven to 200°C/400°F. Line the base of a medium-sized oven dish with baking paper.

Heat the ghee/oil in a pan over a medium/low heat. When the pan is hot, add the sweet potato and onion. Fry gently for 6 minutes, stirring occasionally until soft.

Crack the eggs into a jug. Add the cheese, milk, apple cider vinegar, kale, mustard, sweet potato, and onion.

Bake for 30-35 minutes or until the centre is firm. Cut into four pieces and serve.

Store any leftovers in an airtight container and refrigerate for up to 3 days or freeze on same day.

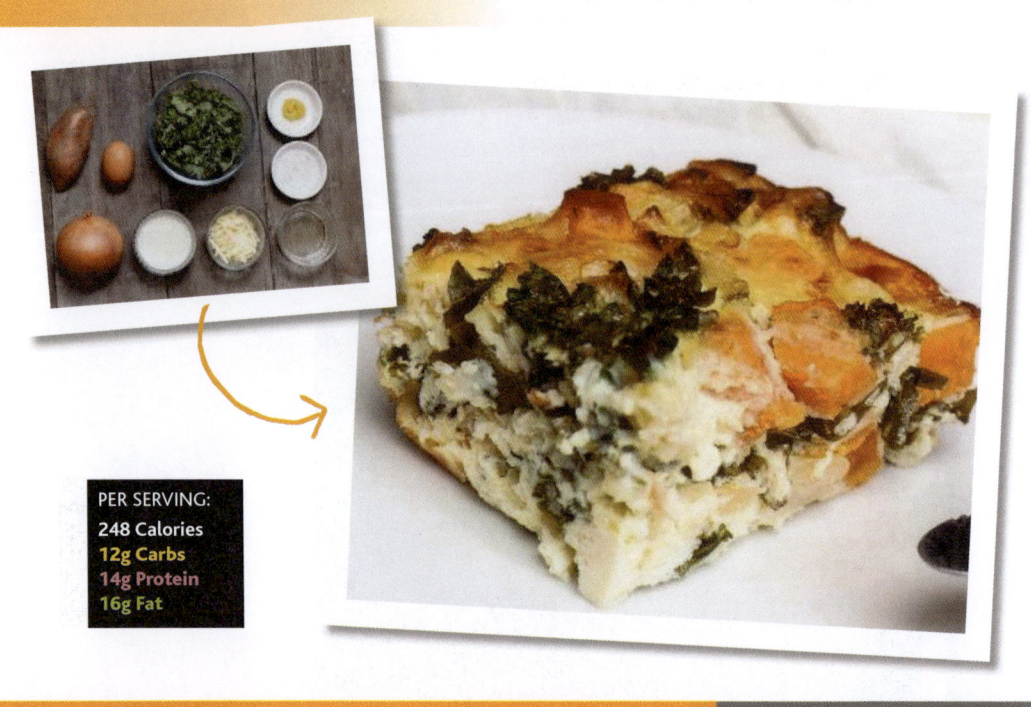

PER SERVING:
248 Calories
12g Carbs
14g Protein
16g Fat

https://thehealthandfitnesscoach.co.uk

LUNCH

Lentil, cucumber & red pepper salad

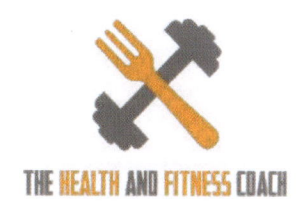

THE HEALTH AND FITNESS COACH

250g (dry weight) red or green lentils
1 red bell-pepper, diced
2 large cucumbers, diced
½ large red onion, finely chopped
1 tbsp fresh parsley, chopped
30ml white wine vinegar
½ tsp sea salt
½ tsp ground black pepper
juice of ½ a lemon
a handful of green olives
½ tsp crushed red chilli flakes

SERVES 4

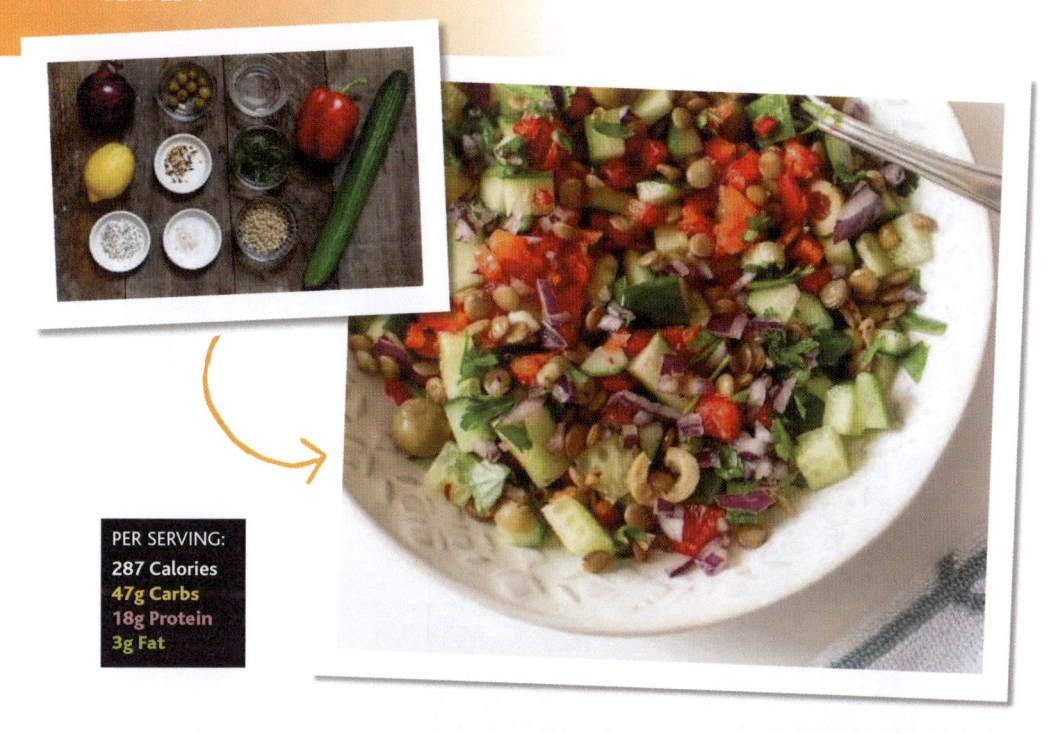

Rinse the lentils in cold water. Place them in a saucepan and cover with cold water. Bring to a boil then reduce heat to simmer. Stir and cook for 25-30 minutes, or until tender.

Drain the lentils and rinse well under cold running water.

Place all of the ingredients in a large bowl and stir well.

Transfer to four bowls and serve.

Store any leftovers in an airtight container and refrigerate for up to 2 days.

PER SERVING:
287 Calories
47g Carbs
18g Protein
3g Fat

https://thehealthandfitnesscoach.co.uk   LUNCH   64

Lemon cod fillets

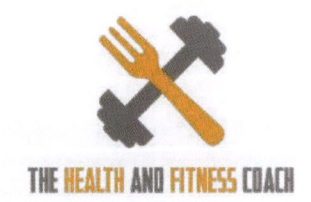

60g ground almonds
2 tsps dried mixed herbs
2 tsps dried chives
1 tsp sea salt
½ tsp ground black pepper
1 tsp garlic granules
4 x 200g cod fillets
4 tbsps butter
juice of 1-2 lemons

SERVES 4

Place the ground almonds, mixed herbs, chives, salt, pepper, and garlic granules in a bowl. Stir well.

Press each cod fillet into the flour mixture, ensuring they are evenly coated on each side.

In a large frying pan, heat 2 tbsps butter over a medium/high heat. When the pan is hot, place two of the cod fillets into the pan using a fish slice.

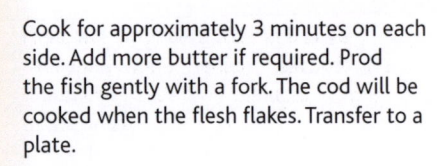

Cook for approximately 3 minutes on each side. Add more butter if required. Prod the fish gently with a fork. The cod will be cooked when the flesh flakes. Transfer to a plate.

Repeat step with the remaining butter and cod fillets.

Squeeze lemon juice over the cod and serve.

Store any leftovers in an airtight container and refrigerate for up to 3 days.

Serving suggestion:

Serve with a mixed salad.

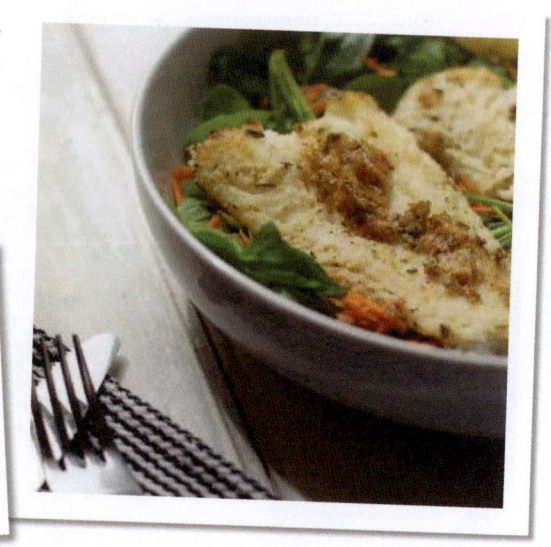

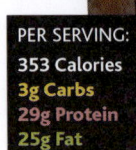

PER SERVING:
353 Calories
3g Carbs
29g Protein
25g Fat

https://thehealthandfitnesscoach.co.uk

LUNCH

Tuna stuffed courgette boats

3 small courgettes, cut in half lengthways
2 tbsps coconut oil or ghee, melted
1 medium-sized white onion, diced
1 garlic clove, minced
½ tsp sea salt
½ tsp ground black pepper
1 tsp dried mixed herbs
100ml cold water
200g tinned chopped tomatoes
150g tinned tuna, drained
50g mature Cheddar cheese, grated
1 tbsp fresh parsley, finely chopped

SERVES 2

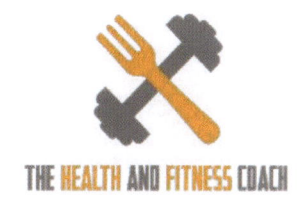

Preheat oven to 180°C/350°F. Gently score the skin of each courgette in a criss-cross pattern. Carefully scoop out the flesh from each courgette and roughly chop.

Drizzle 1 tbsp oil/ghee into the base of a large rectangular ovenproof dish. Place the courgette halves in the dish, skin side facing down.

Heat the remaining oil/ghee in a frying pan over a medium heat. Add the onion and courgette flesh. Fry gently until the onion is soft and translucent. Add the garlic and fry for 2 minutes, stirring occasionally.

Add the salt, pepper, mixed herbs, water, and tinned tomatoes. Stir well and cook for 3 minutes, stirring occasionally until the sauce begins to reduce.

Add the tuna and stir well. Remove the pan from the heat. Spoon the mixture into each courgette. Sprinkle with cheese.

Bake for 25 minutes. Serve garnished with fresh parsley.

Store any leftovers in an airtight container and refrigerate for up to 1 day.

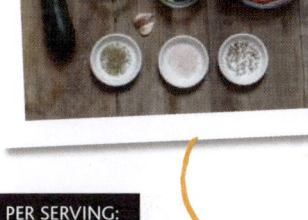

PER SERVING:
417 Calories
16g Carbs
32g Protein
25g Fat

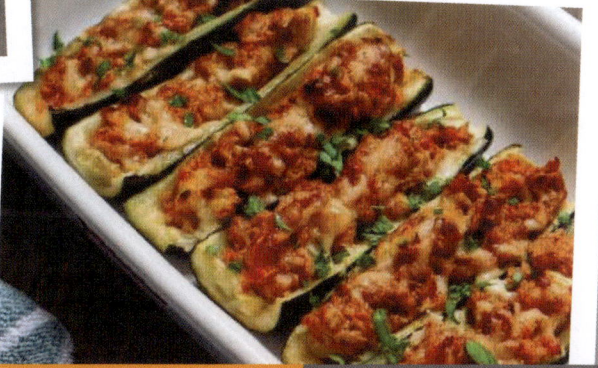

https://thehealthandfitnesscoach.co.uk

Chicken lentil soup

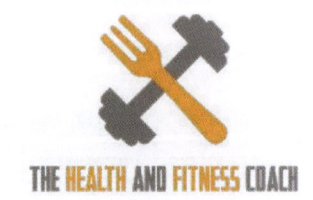

4 tbsps coconut oil, butter or ghee
1 large white onion, diced
3 garlic cloves, thinly sliced
2 medium-sized celery stalks, sliced
2 medium-sized carrots, sliced
½ tsp sea salt
½ tsp ground black pepper
2 tbsps tomato purée
2 litres vegetable stock (made with 1½ organic stock cubes)
80g green or red dried lentils, rinsed and drained
1lb chicken breast or thigh fillet, finely diced

SERVES 8

Heat the oil/ghee/butter in a large saucepan over a medium heat. Add the onion and sauté for 4 minutes, stirring occasionally.

Add the garlic, celery, carrots, salt and pepper. Cook over a medium/low heat for 8-10 minutes, stirring occasionally.

Add the tomato purée and stir. Add the vegetable stock and lentils. Increase heat and bring to a boil then reduce heat to simmer gently.

Add the chicken. Cover and cook for 45 minutes to 1 hour. Stir occasionally and add more stock during cooking time, if required. Serve.

Store any leftovers in an airtight container and refrigerate for up to 3 days, or freeze on same day.

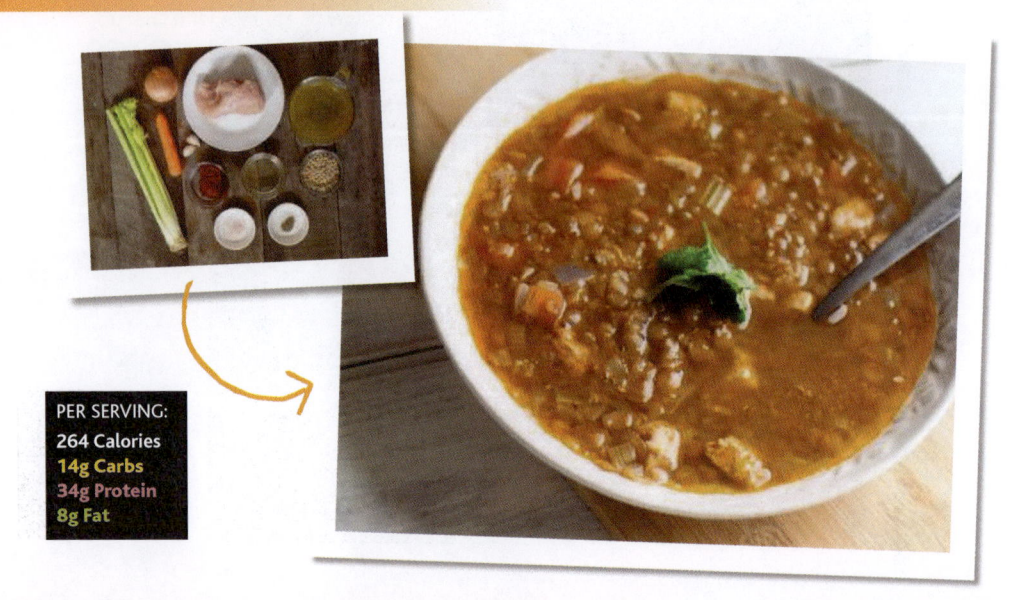

PER SERVING:
264 Calories
14g Carbs
34g Protein
8g Fat

https://thehealthandfitnesscoach.co.uk

LUNCH 67

Dijon chicken wings

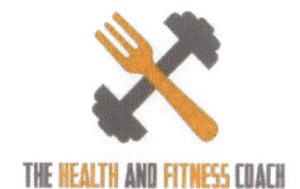

5lb chicken wings
1 tbsp olive oil
1 tbsp tomato purée
1 medium-sized white onion, finely sliced
2 garlic cloves, minced
½ tbsp mixed herbs
½ tbsp ground coriander
½ tsp paprika
½ tsp ground black pepper
½ tsp sea salt
1 tbsp Dijon mustard
1 tsp honey
2 spring onions, finely sliced

SERVES 8

Line 2 baking trays with foil.

Place the chicken in a large bowl. Add the olive oil, tomato purée, onion, garlic, spices, mustard and honey.

Cover with cling film and marinate in the fridge for 1 hour.

Remove from the refrigerator and leave at room temperature for 10 minutes.

Meanwhile, preheat oven to 200°C/400°F.

Place the chicken wings onto the baking trays. Cover loosely with foil and bake for 30 minutes.

Remove the foil and cook for another 15-20 minutes, or until cooked.

Garnish with spring onions and serve.

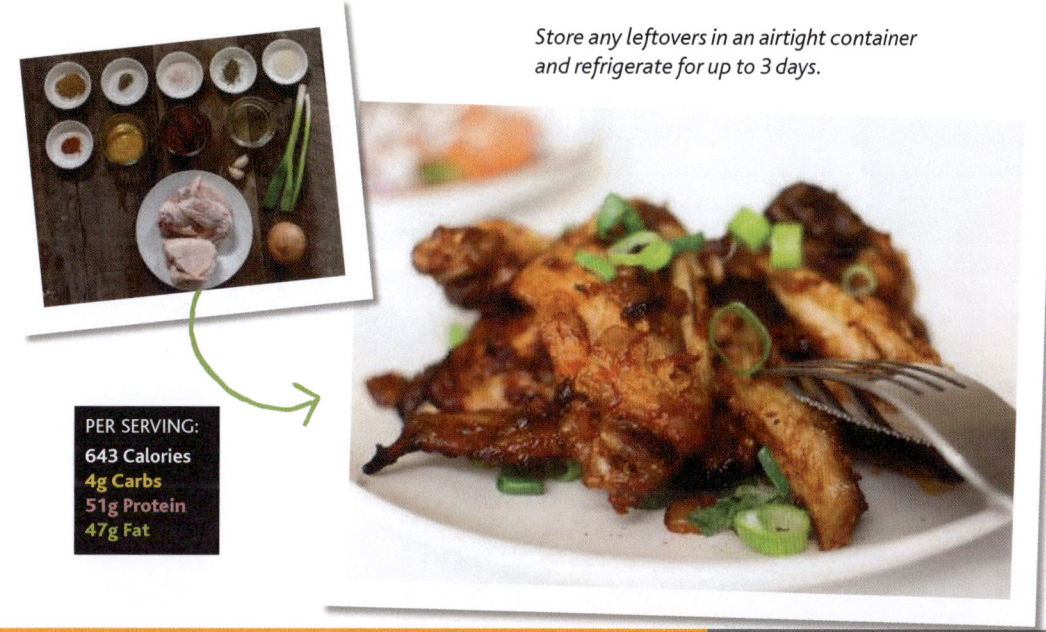

Store any leftovers in an airtight container and refrigerate for up to 3 days.

PER SERVING:
643 Calories
4g Carbs
51g Protein
47g Fat

Shish tawook

900g fresh chicken breast, diced

for the marinade:
juice of ½ a lemon
65g plain yoghurt (use dairy free if preferred)
2 tbsps olive oil
2 tbsps tomato purée
2 tsps paprika
1 tsp ground black pepper
1 tsp dried thyme or mixed herbs
1 tsp cayenne pepper
3 garlic cloves, minced

SERVES 4

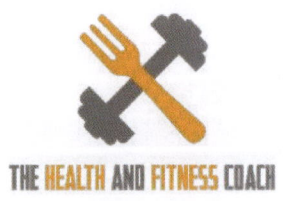

Place the marinade ingredients in a large bowl and stir well.

Add the chicken and stir well. Cover with cling film and refrigerate for 3 hours, or overnight if you have time.

Soak 8 wooden skewers in cold water for 30 minutes, or prepare 8 metal skewers.

Preheat oven to 180°C/350°F. Line a baking tray with foil.

Thread the chicken onto the skewers. Place the skewers onto the baking tray.

Bake for 10 minutes, then turn and cook for another 10 minutes, or until golden and thoroughly cooked.

Store any leftovers in an airtight container and refrigerate for up to 2 days.

Serving suggestion:
Serve with salad and steamed rice.

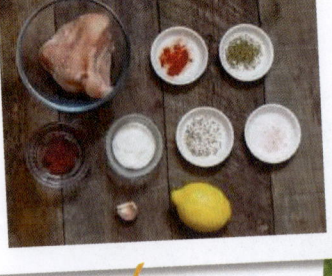

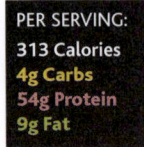

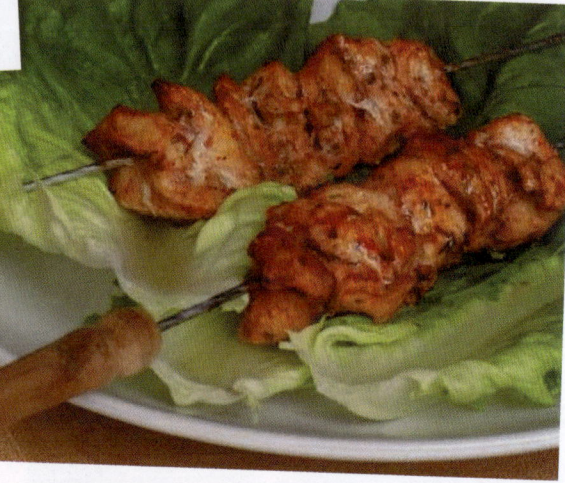

PER SERVING:
313 Calories
4g Carbs
54g Protein
9g Fat

https://thehealthandfitnesscoach.co.uk

Chicken bulgur salad

100g bulgur wheat (uncooked weight), rinsed
200ml recently boiled water
400g fresh chicken breast
2 tbsps olive oil
1 tsp sea salt
1 tsp ground black pepper
½ tsp paprika
1 ripe salad tomato, diced
1 large cucumber, sliced
50g romaine lettuce, shredded
30g pitted olives (any colour)
50g fresh spinach leaves
2 tbsps fresh parsley, finely chopped
50g Feta cheese
juice of ½ a lemon

SERVES 4

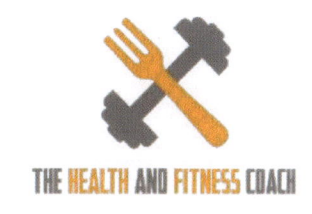

Line a baking tray with foil.

Place the bulgur wheat in a large bowl and add the boiled water. Cover the bowl with cling film. Set aside for 30 minutes.

Brush the chicken breast with 1 tbsp olive oil and season with half of the salt and pepper.

Place the chicken onto the baking tray and bake for 25-30 minutes, or until the juices run clear.

Place the paprika and the remaining oil, salt and pepper in a large bowl.

Place the tomato, cucumber, lettuce, olives, spinach and parsley in a large bowl. Slice or shred the chicken breast into the bowl. Add the cheese, bulgur wheat and lemon juice and mix well.

Divide between four serving bowls. Serve.

Store any leftovers in an airtight container and refrigerate for up to 2 days.

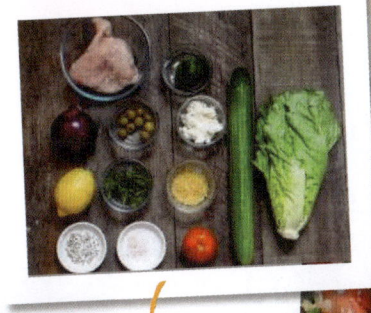

PER SERVING:
337 Calories
27g Carbs
28g Protein
13g Fat

https://thehealthandfitnesscoach.co.uk

Lentil kibbeh

200g red lentils (uncooked weight)
340g bulgur wheat
1 tsp coconut oil
1 medium-sized red onion, diced
1 red bell-pepper, diced
1 tsp sea salt
2 tbsps tomato purée
½ tsp cayenne pepper
1 tsp paprika
1 tsp ground cumin
3 tbsps cold water
500g romaine lettuce

to serve:
120g plain yoghurt (use dairy free if preferred)

SERVES 6

Pour 700ml recently boiled water into a saucepan. Place over a medium/high heat and bring to a boil. Add the lentils and cook for 8 minutes.

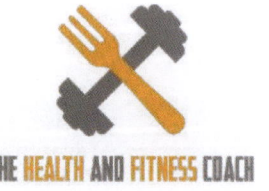

Reduce the heat to low and add the bulgur wheat. Cover and cook for 15 minutes, stirring occasionally. When the water has absorbed and the bulgur wheat is cooked, remove the pan from the heat and set aside to cool.

Melt the coconut oil in a saucepan over a medium heat. Add the onion, bell-pepper, salt, tomato purée, cayenne pepper, paprika and cumin. Cook for 2 minutes, stirring occasionally. Add the cold water and stir well. Transfer to a large bowl and add the cooked lentils and bulgur wheat. Stir well.

Preheat oven to 200°C/400°F. Line two baking trays with baking paper.

Scoop out 2 tbsps of the mixture, roll into a ball and flatten gently. Place onto the baking tray. Repeat with the remaining mixture. Ensure the balls are spaced at least 2cm apart on the tray. Bake for 20 minutes, or until golden.

Arrange the romaine lettuce leaves onto a plate and place the kibbehs on top. Drizzle the yoghurt over the top and serve.

Store any leftover kibbehs in an airtight container and refrigerate for up to 3 days or freeze on same day.

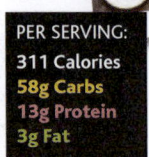

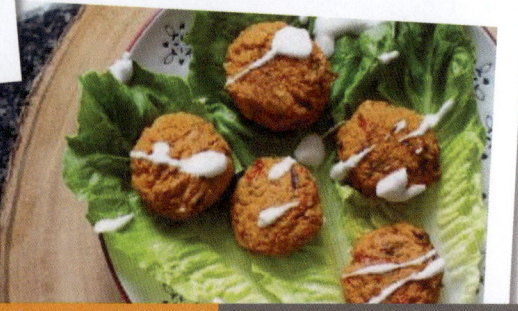

PER SERVING:
311 Calories
58g Carbs
13g Protein
3g Fat

https://thehealthandfitnesscoach.co.uk

LUNCH

Bulgur & butternut squash bowl

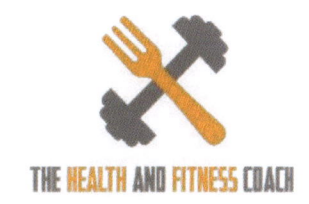

190g bulgur wheat
200ml cold water
1 small butternut squash, deseeded and cubed
1 red bell-pepper, left whole
1 tbsp olive oil
1 tsp coconut oil
170g fresh spinach leaves
2 tsps sesame oil
¼ tsp ground black pepper
¼ tsp sea salt
3 tbsps soy sauce or tamari
40g pine nuts

SERVES 4

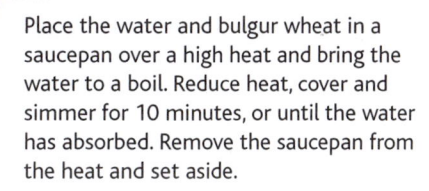

Place the water and bulgur wheat in a saucepan over a high heat and bring the water to a boil. Reduce heat, cover and simmer for 10 minutes, or until the water has absorbed. Remove the saucepan from the heat and set aside.

Preheat oven to 180°C/350°F. Line a baking tray with baking paper.

Place the squash and bell-pepper onto the tray and toss with the olive oil. Bake for 20 minutes or until soft, turning the pepper several times during cooking time.

Heat the coconut oil in a saucepan over a medium heat. Add the spinach and cook for two minutes, or until the spinach has wilted. Remove the pan from the heat.

When the pepper is cool enough to handle, remove the stem and seeds and discard. Chop the pepper into chunks.

Place the sesame oil, black pepper, salt, bulgur wheat, soy sauce, spinach, butternut squash and red bell-pepper in a large bowl. Toss the ingredients and sprinkle the pine nuts over the top. Serve.

Store any leftovers in an airtight container and refrigerate for up to 2 days.

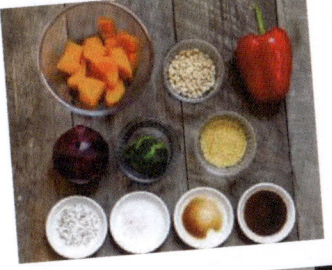

PER SERVING:
442 Calories
67g Carbs
12g Protein
14g Fat

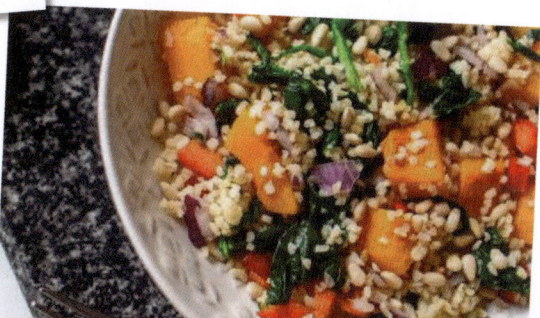

https://thehealthandfitnesscoach.co.uk

LUNCH

Vegan scalloped potatoes

1 tsp coconut oil or olive oil
150ml hot vegetable stock (made with one organic stock cube)
200ml unsweetened almond milk
2 tbsps corn flour or rice flour
1 tsp garlic powder
1 tsp onion powder
a small pinch of ground nutmeg
1 tsp paprika
a small pinch of cayenne pepper
1 tsp dried mixed herbs
5 tbsps nutritional yeast
3 medium-sized white potatoes, cut into 1cm thick slices
½ tsp sea salt
2 tbsps fresh parsley, finely chopped

SERVES 2

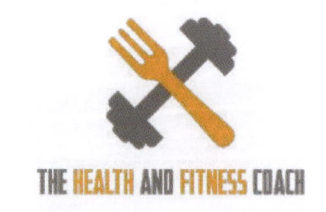

Preheat oven to 200°C/400°F. Lightly grease an ovenproof dish with oil.

Pour the stock and milk into a saucepan. Add the corn flour, dried spices and nutritional yeast.

Place the saucepan over a medium heat. Bring to a simmer and cook for five minutes, whisking continuously.

Arrange the potatoes around the base of the dish and season with salt. Pour the stock over the potatoes.

Cover with foil and bake for 20 minutes. Remove the foil and bake for 30-40 minutes, or until cooked to your liking.

Allow to stand for five minutes, sprinkle over the parsley, and serve.

Store any leftovers in an airtight container and refrigerate for up to 3 days or freeze on same day.

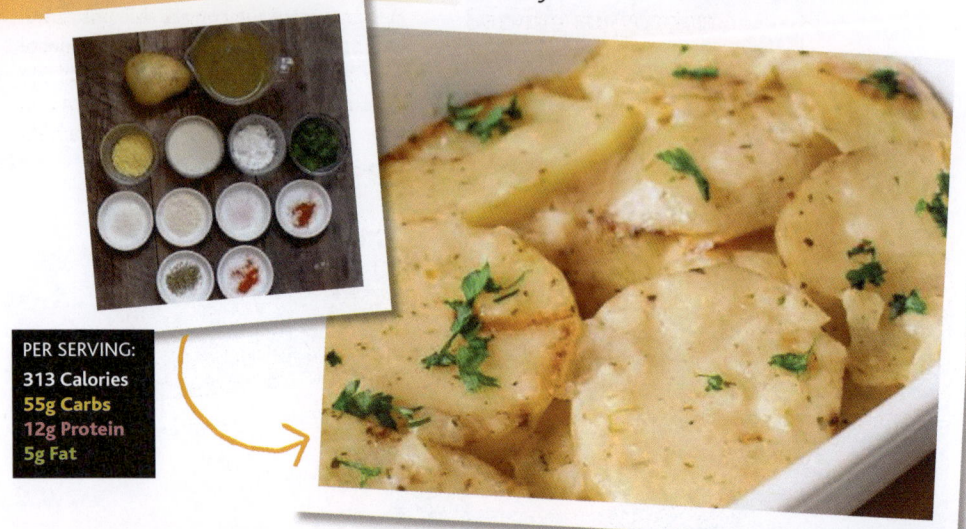

PER SERVING:
313 Calories
55g Carbs
12g Protein
5g Fat

https://thehealthandfitnesscoach.co.uk

LUNCH

Caprese chicken salad

for the dressing:
15ml balsamic vinegar
2 tsps olive oil
¼ tsp dried basil
a small pinch of sea salt

for the salad:
100g cooked roast chicken, skin removed and shredded
1 romaine lettuce, washed and sliced
50g ripe avocado, sliced
3 vine-ripened tomatoes, halved
20g Mozzarella cheese, torn into small pieces
3-5 basil leaves
a small pinch of ground black pepper

SERVES 1

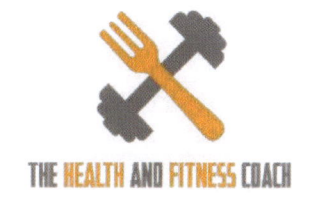

Mix the dressing ingredients in a jug.

Place the lettuce leaves in a serving bowl.

Assemble the remaining salad ingredients over the lettuce.

Drizzle the dressing over the salad. Serve.

Store any leftovers in an airtight container and refrigerate for up to 1 day.

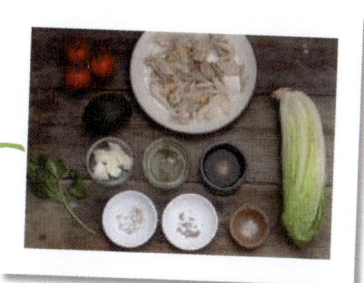

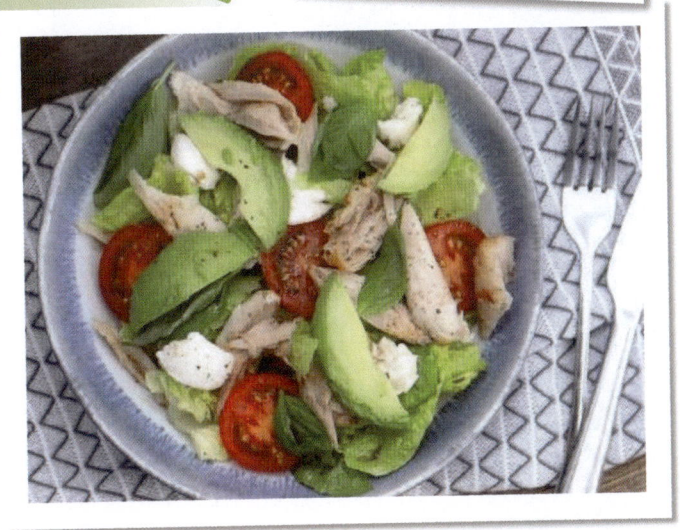

PER SERVING:
453 Calories
10g Carbs
38g Protein
29g Fat

https://thehealthandfitnesscoach.co.uk   LUNCH   74

Garlic & herb roast chicken

2kg whole chicken (giblets removed)
2 tbsps olive oil
25g unsalted butter, at room temperature, cut into large pieces
1-2 tsps sea salt, to taste
1-2 tsps ground black pepper, to taste
4 garlic cloves, peeled and minced
1 head of garlic, peeled, half minced, half left whole
3 rosemary sprigs
1 lemon
2 tbsps parsley, finely chopped
1 tbsp dried parsley
1 tsp dried thyme

SERVES 5

Preheat oven to 200°C /400°F. Prepare a roasting dish. Using your hands, gently loosen the skin from the surface of the chicken. Start from the breast near the neck and move carefully over the surface of the chicken.

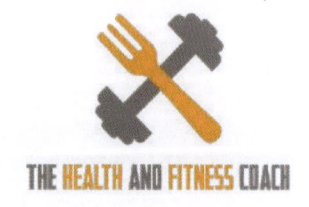

Place the pieces of butter under the skin, distributing around the chicken. Drizzle the olive oil over the chicken. Season with salt and pepper. Sprinkle the minced garlic over the chicken.

Stuff the remaining garlic into the chicken cavity along with the rosemary sprigs. Pierce the lemon twice using a skewer and place in the chicken cavity.

Tie the legs together with twine. Place the chicken into the roasting dish. Roast for 1 hour 20 minutes, basting half way through cooking time.

At the end of cooking time, baste again and roast for 5 minutes. Remove from the oven, cover with foil and allow to stand for 10 minutes before serving. Pour the juices over the chicken. Serve.

Store any leftover chicken in an airtight container and refrigerate for up to 2 days.

Serving suggestion:

Halfway through cooking time, add some chopped root vegetables around the base of the chicken. Stir to cover in the juices

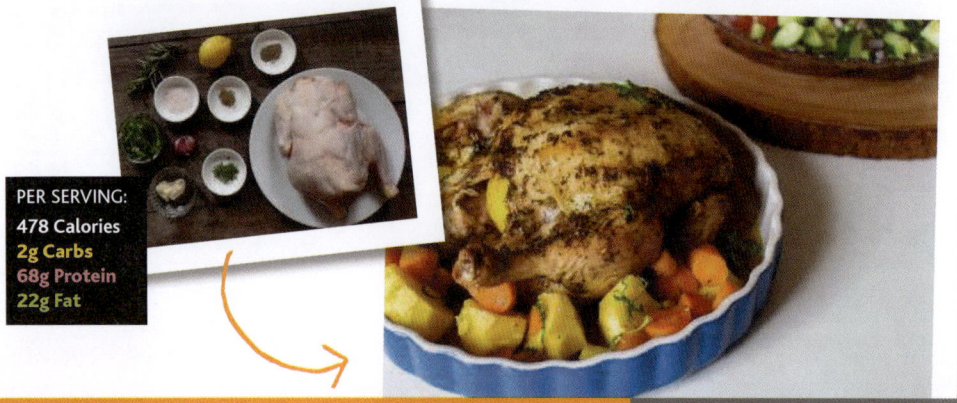

PER SERVING:
478 Calories
2g Carbs
68g Protein
22g Fat

https://thehealthandfitnesscoach.co.uk

DINNER

Chicken in a creamy leek sauce

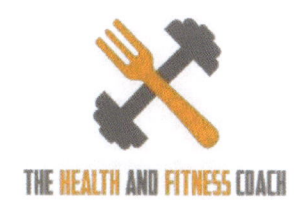

1 heaped tsp ghee or coconut oil
2 x 200g chicken breasts
½ a medium-sized white onion, finely chopped
1 garlic clove, crushed
130g closed cup mushrooms, sliced
1 medium-sized leek, finely sliced
250ml chicken stock (made with one organic stock cube)
a pinch of sea salt and ground black pepper
a large handful of spinach leaves
30ml crème fraîche
1 tbsp fresh parsley, finely chopped

SERVES 2

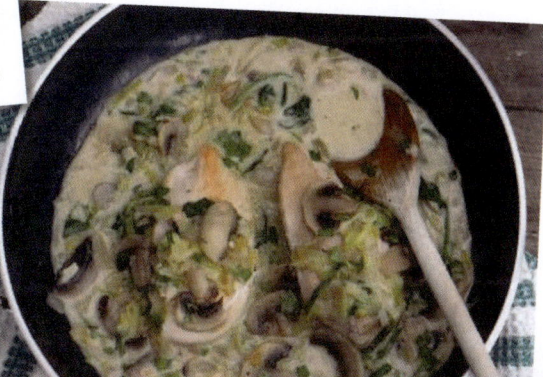

Heat half of the ghee/oil in a frying pan over a medium heat. Add the chicken breasts and fry for 10 minutes, or until well browned on both sides. Transfer to a plate and set aside.

Add the remaining ghee/oil and fry the onion for 2–3 minutes, stirring occasionally until soft. Add the garlic and fry for 1–2 minutes, stirring occasionally. Add the mushrooms and leek and fry for 4-5 minutes, stirring occasionally.

Return the chicken to the pan and stir in the stock. Bring to the boil then reduce heat to simmer. Cover and cook for 10 minutes, or until the chicken is cooked.

Stir in the salt and pepper. Add the spinach and cook until wilted. Stir in the crème fraîche and parsley and serve.

Store any leftovers in an airtight container and refrigerate for up to 3 days or freeze on same day.

Serving suggestion:

Serve with steamed rice or over toasted sourdough

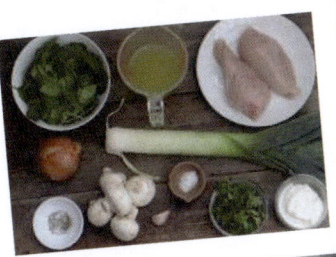

PER SERVING:
399 Calories
17g Carbs
49g Protein
15g Fat

https://thehealthandfitnesscoach.co.uk

DINNER

Pan fried coconut & chilli fish with a spinach salad

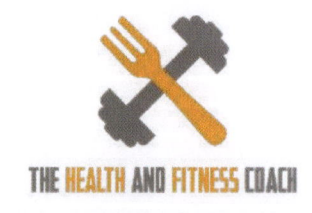

300g halibut steaks or firm white fish
1 heaped tbsp desiccated coconut
1 tbsp plain flour (use gluten free if preferred)
lemon slices, to serve
2 tbsps coconut oil

for the salad:
a handful of spinach leaves
160g cucumber, diced
1 red bell-pepper, diced
1 vine-ripened tomato, finely diced
1 tbsp fresh coriander, finely chopped
a pinch of sea salt
2 tbsps fresh lemon juice

for the marinade:
1 red chilli pepper
1 tsp fresh ginger, peeled
a small bunch of fresh parsley
3 garlic cloves, peeled
2 tsps white wine vinegar
1 tsp ground coriander
a pinch of sea salt and black pepper

SERVES 2

PER SERVING:
402 Calories
21g Carbs
39g Protein
18g Fat

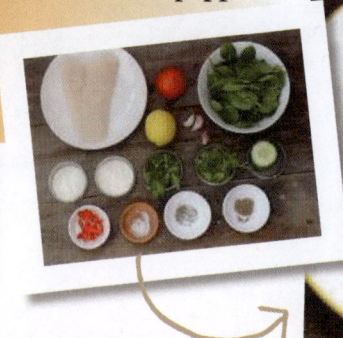

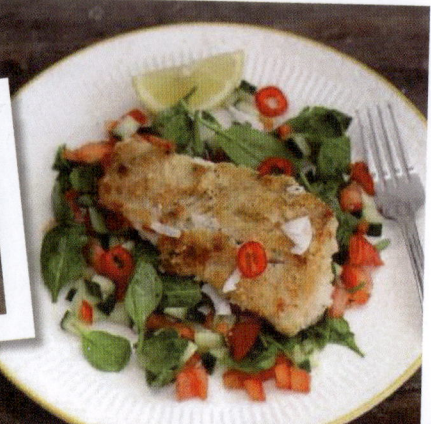

Mix the salad ingredients in a bowl. Using a wooden spoon, pound the spinach leaves gently. Cover and refrigerate.

Meanwhile, place the marinade ingredients in a blender and blend well until smooth.

Place the fish in a bowl and pour over the marinade. Stir to coat the fish. Cover and refrigerate for 30 minutes (or longer if you have time).

Mix the coconut and flour together in a shallow based bowl. Add the fish and cover both sides in the mixture.

Melt the oil in a frying pan over a low heat. Add the fish and cook for 3 minutes. Avoid touching the fish while it cooks. Turn with a slice and cook for 3 minutes, or until the fish is cooked. Serve the fish over a bed of spinach salad.

Store any leftovers in an airtight container and refrigerate for up to 1 day.

THE HEALTH AND FITNESS COACH

https://thehealthandfitnesscoach.co.uk

DINNER 77

Greek lamb chops

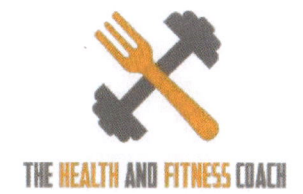

9 lamb chops, visible fat removed
for the marinade:
25g butter, softened
2 tsps dried oregano
3 garlic cloves, minced
1 tsp dried parsley
1 tsp sea salt
½ tsp freshly ground black pepper
for the garnish:
a sprinkle of fresh parsley, chopped

SERVES 3

Pat the lamb chops dry using kitchen roll.

Place the marinade ingredients in a wide-based bowl and stir well. Add the lamb.

Rub the marinade into the lamb chops. Cover and refrigerate for 30 minutes or longer if time. Allow the lamb chops to rest for 10 minutes at room temperature before cooking.

Place a large frying pan over a medium heat. Add the lamb chops and fry for 3 minutes on each side for medium cooked. Cook for a little less time if you prefer medium/rare, or a little longer if you prefer well done.

Allow the lamb chops to rest for 5 minutes before serving. Serve garnished with parsley.

Store any leftover cooked lamb chops in an airtight container and refrigerate for up to 2 days. Any uncooked lamb chops can be frozen on the same day.

Serving suggestion:
Serve with steamed rice and salad or steamed vegetables

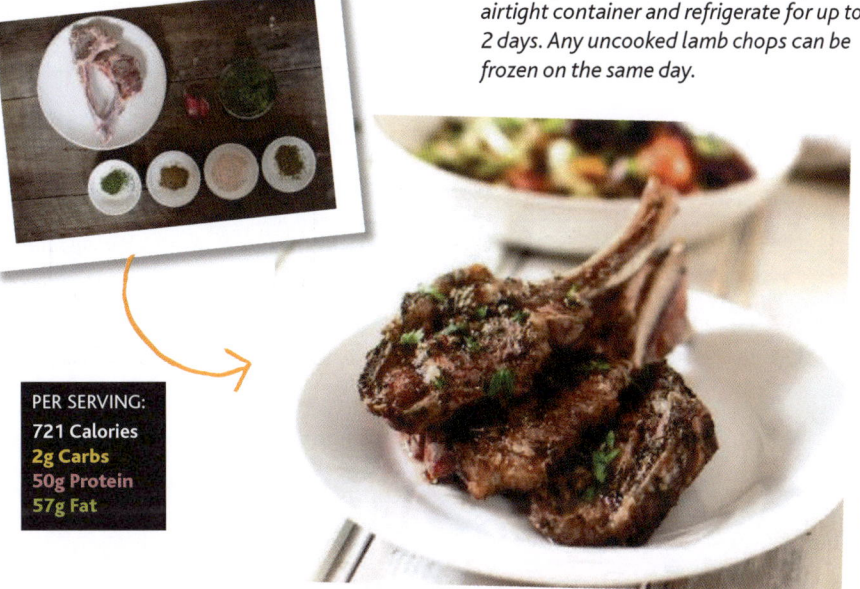

PER SERVING:
721 Calories
2g Carbs
50g Protein
57g Fat

https://thehealthandfitnesscoach.co.uk

Vegetarian moussaka

160g brown lentils (uncooked)
600g white potatoes, peeled
1 tsp coconut oil
2 medium-sized white onions, finely chopped
2 garlic cloves, finely chopped
4 sprigs fresh thyme (leaves only)
½ tsp dried oregano
½ tsp ground cinnamon
1 tbsp tomato purée
400g tinned chopped tomatoes
1 organic vegetable stock cube
½ tsp sea salt
1 tsp ground black pepper
2 large aubergines, thinly sliced
225g ricotta cheese (use dairy free cheese if preferred)
55g mature Cheddar, grated (use dairy free cheese if preferred)
2 tbsps fresh parsley, chopped

SERVES 5

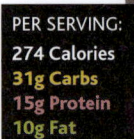

Preheat oven to 200°C/400°F. Soak the lentils in cold water and set aside. Place the potatoes into a large saucepan. Cover with water then bring to the boil. Reduce heat and simmer for 15 minutes, or until fork-tender. Drain and set aside.

Heat the oil in a saucepan over a medium heat. Add the onions and fry for 5 minutes, stirring occasionally until soft. Add the garlic, thyme, oregano, cinnamon and tomato purée and cook for 1 minute.

Add the tomatoes, salt and pepper and 800ml recently boiled water. Crumble in the stock cube. Drain the lentils then add to the saucepan. Stir and simmer for 20 minutes, or until the lentils are tender.

Heat a skillet until hot, then griddle the aubergine until brown and slightly soft. Slice the potatoes (approximately 5mm thickness). Pour half of the lentil sauce into a medium-sized oven dish then layer half the potatoes and aubergines over the top. Add the remaining lentils, potatoes and aubergines.

Top with the cheese. Bake for 25 minutes, or until golden brown. Garnish with parsley.

Store any leftovers in an airtight container and refrigerate for up to 3 days or freeze on same day.

PER SERVING:
274 Calories
31g Carbs
15g Protein
10g Fat

https://thehealthandfitnesscoach.co.uk

DINNER

Beef & lentil stew

1 tbsp olive oil
1 large white onion, chopped
250g celery, chopped
3 medium-sized carrots, chopped
3 garlic cloves, chopped
1kg beef, cubed
1 litre vegetable stock (made with one organic stock cube)
2 bay leaves
½ tsp cayenne pepper
1 tbsp mixed herbs
sea salt, to taste
ground black pepper, to taste
400g tomatoes (canned or diced)
150g green lentils (uncooked), rinsed

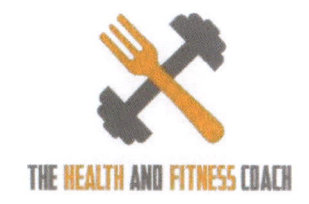

SERVES 8

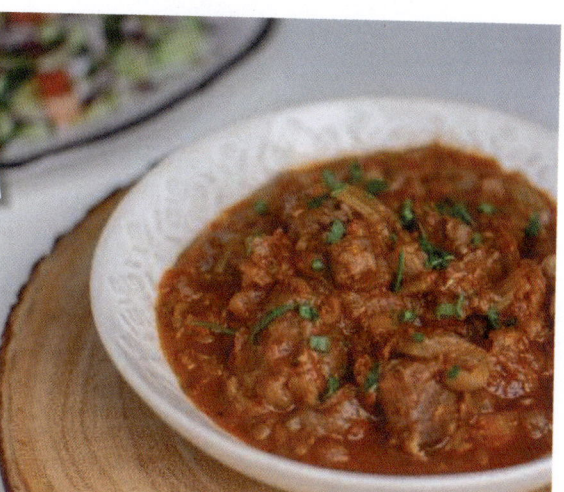

Heat the oil in a large saucepan over a medium heat. Add the onion, carrots and celery and sauté for 5 minutes, stirring occasionally until soft and translucent.

Add the garlic and fry for one minute, stirring occasionally.

Add the beef and fry for 8 minutes, stirring occasionally to ensure all sides are browned.

Add the stock, bay leaves, herbs and spices, tomatoes and lentils.

Bring to the boil then reduce the heat to simmer. Cover and cook for one hour. Serve.

Store any leftovers in an airtight container and refrigerate for up to 3 days or freeze on same day.

Serving suggestion:

Serve with a mixed salad or steamed vegetables of your choice

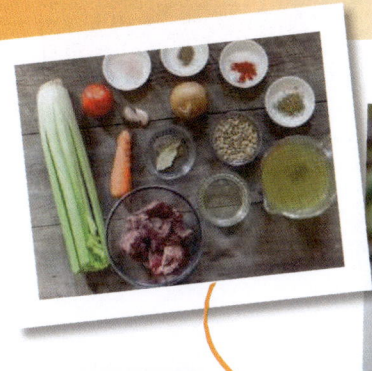

PER SERVING:
279 Calories
15g Carbs
30g Protein
11g Fat

https://thehealthandfitnesscoach.co.uk

DINNER

Chicken & vegetable pizza

9g instant yeast
1 tsp honey
420g all purpose flour (use gluten free if preferred)
2½ tsps xanthan gum
½ tsp sea salt
85ml olive oil
250ml cold water
100g cooked chicken breast, diced
1 tbsp tomato purée
60g mozzarella cheese, grated
1 bell-pepper (any colour), chopped
100g button mushrooms, chopped
2 tsps dried mixed herbs
½ tsp ground black pepper
½ tsp sea salt
50g pitted olives (any colour), sliced

SERVES 4

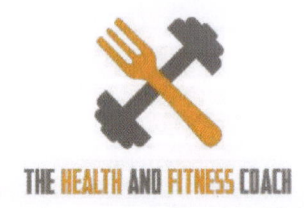

Lightly grease the base of a baking tin. Transfer the dough into the tin. Cover with cling film and place a tea towel on top. Allow to sit for 1 hour in a warm environment. Refrigerate the dough for 20 minutes.

Preheat oven to 200°C/400°F. Lightly flour a clean surface and roll out the dough into a large circle, moving the dough occasionally so that it doesn't stick to the surface. Using your fingertips, press in the dough, 1 inch from the edge to create a crust. Brush lightly with olive oil.

Place a frying pan over a medium heat and add the remaining olive oil. Add the diced chicken breast, toss and cook for 2 minutes.

Bake the pizza dough for 3 minutes. Spread the tomato purée over the base. Add the remaining toppings. Bake for 5-10 minutes, or until browned. Cut into 4 pieces.

Store any leftovers in an airtight container and refrigerate for up to 3 days or freeze on same day.

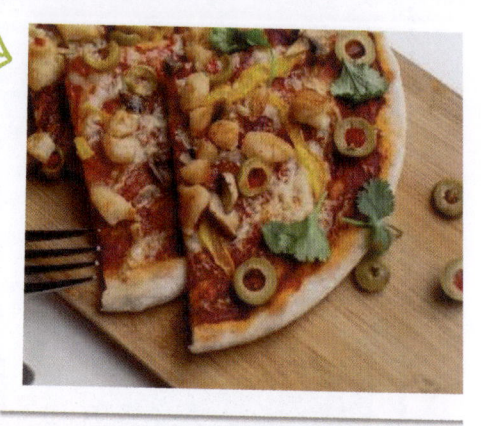

In a small bowl mix together the yeast and honey. In a separate large bowl mix the flour, xanthan gum and salt. Make a well in the centre. Pour 70ml olive oil, cold water and yeast mixture into the well. Mix well and knead for 5 minutes.

PER SERVING:
480 Calories
78g Carbs
24g Protein
8g Fat

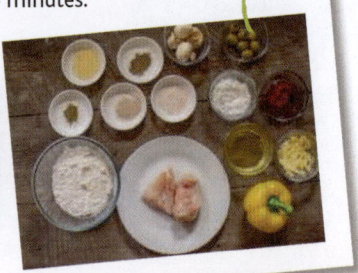

https://thehealthandfitnesscoach.co.uk

DINNER

Roast cauliflower chicken

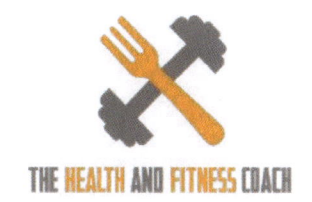

6 skinless chicken thighs
½ tsp sea salt
¼ tsp ground black pepper
1 tbsp dried mixed herbs
1 tbsp fresh rosemary
6 cloves garlic, minced
40g butter
½ a large cauliflower head, cut into florets
juice of 1 lemon

SERVES 3

Preheat oven to 190°C/375°F.

Season the chicken thighs with salt, pepper, mixed herbs, rosemary and garlic.

Melt the butter in a frying pan over a medium heat.

Place the chicken thighs in a large roasting tin and pour over the butter. Arrange the cauliflower florets around the chicken.

Roast for 40 minutes, or until the chicken is cooked.

Squeeze the lemon juice over the chicken and serve.

Store any leftovers in an airtight container and refrigerate for up to 4 days or freeze on same day.

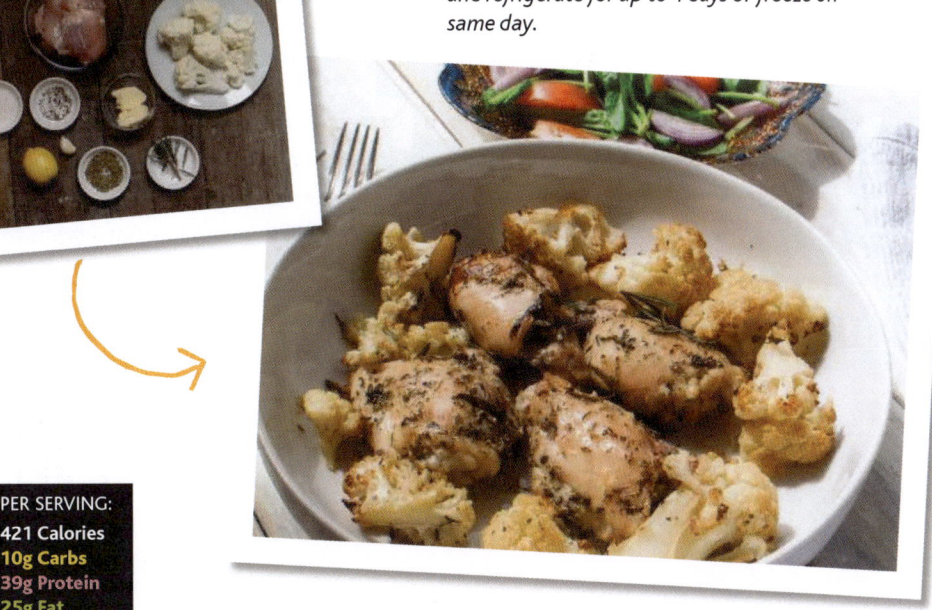

PER SERVING:
421 Calories
10g Carbs
39g Protein
25g Fat

Mongolian beef

30g corn starch or rice flour
300g beef flank steak, sliced into ½ inch thick pieces
30ml coconut or olive oil
1 tbsp fresh ginger, minced
1 tbsp fresh garlic, minced
30ml soy sauce or tamari
60ml cold water
30ml honey
4 spring onions, sliced

SERVES 2

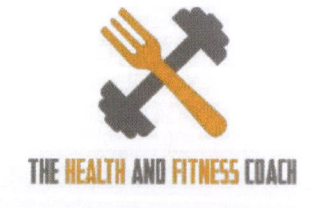

Place the corn starch in a plastic food bag or sealable container. Add the steak pieces and shake gently, ensuring the pieces are well coated.

Heat the oil in a large frying pan over a medium/high heat. Add the steak pieces (in batches if preferred), gently shaking off any excess corn starch before placing them in the pan. Fry for 2 minutes on each side. Transfer the cooked steak to a plate and set aside.

Add the ginger and garlic to the frying pan and fry for 15 seconds or until fragrant.

Add the soy sauce, water and honey to the pan and bring to a boil.

Add the steak back into the pan, reduce heat and simmer for 30 seconds. The sauce will thicken as it cooks.

Stir in the spring onions and cook for one minute. Serve.

Store any leftovers in an airtight container and refrigerate for up to 3 days or freeze on same day.

PER SERVING:
309 Calories
15g Carbs
33g Protein
13g Fat

DINNER

Stuffed aubergine

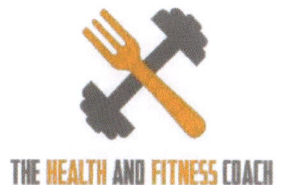

4 large aubergines
3 tsps olive oil
1 tsp sea salt
1 large white onion, finely chopped
250g lean lamb mince
3 garlic cloves, finely chopped
1 tsp dried thyme
¼ tsp chilli flakes
4 small ripe tomatoes, chopped
½ tsp ground black pepper
25g Pecorino cheese (optional), finely grated
3 tbsps fresh basil leaves, thinly sliced

SERVES 4

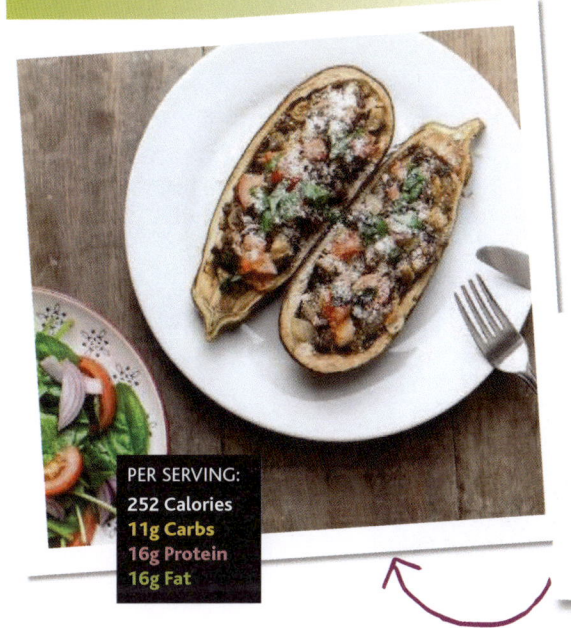

Preheat oven to 200°C/400°F.

Slice each aubergine in half lengthways and scoop out the flesh. Dice the flesh and set aside. Place the aubergine halves in a large roasting dish, flat side facing up.

Brush the inside of the aubergines with a little olive oil and season with a little salt.

Heat 2 tsps olive oil in a pan. Add the onion and fry gently over a medium heat for 6 minutes, stirring occasionally.

Add the lamb mince and stir well, breaking up finely with a wooden spoon as it cooks.

Increase the heat, add the garlic and aubergine flesh. Stir until the flesh is lightly browned. Add the dried thyme, chilli flakes and tomatoes and season with salt and pepper. Stir well and reduce the heat. Cover and simmer for 10 minutes.

Spoon the mixture into the aubergine halves. Drizzle lightly with olive oil. Bake for 20 minutes. Sprinkle over the cheese (if using) and fresh basil and serve.

Store any leftovers in an airtight container and refrigerate for up to 3 days.

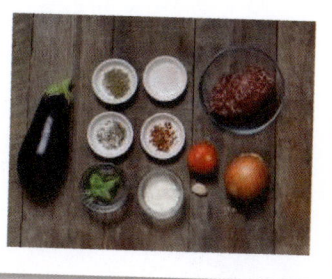

PER SERVING:
252 Calories
11g Carbs
16g Protein
16g Fat

https://thehealthandfitnesscoach.co.uk

DINNER

Lamb curry

2 medium-sized white onions, diced
4 garlic cloves, finely chopped
700ml cold water
2 tbsps ghee or coconut oil
1kg lamb leg, diced
400g tinned chopped tomatoes
½ tbsp fennel seeds
1 tsp barahat or allspice
1 tsp ground coriander
1 tsp ground turmeric
1 tsp ground cumin
1 tsp ground black pepper
1 tsp sea salt
2 green chilli peppers, finely chopped

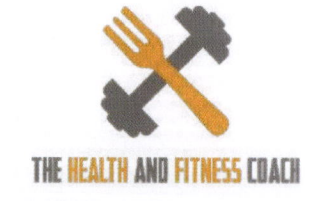

SERVES 5

Place the onions, garlic and 300ml cold water into a food processor and blend until smooth.

Pour into a large saucepan. Cover and simmer for 20 minutes.

Remove the lid and simmer for 5-10 minutes, or until the liquid has fully absorbed.

Melt the ghee/oil in the saucepan. Add the lamb. Fry gently, stirring to brown all over.

Add the tinned tomatoes, remaining cold water, fennel seeds, baharat, coriander, turmeric, salt, pepper and cumin. Simmer for 1 hour 20 minutes, stirring occasionally. Add more water during cooking time, if required.

Add the chilli peppers and serve.

Store any leftovers in an airtight container and refrigerate for up to 3 days or freeze on same day.

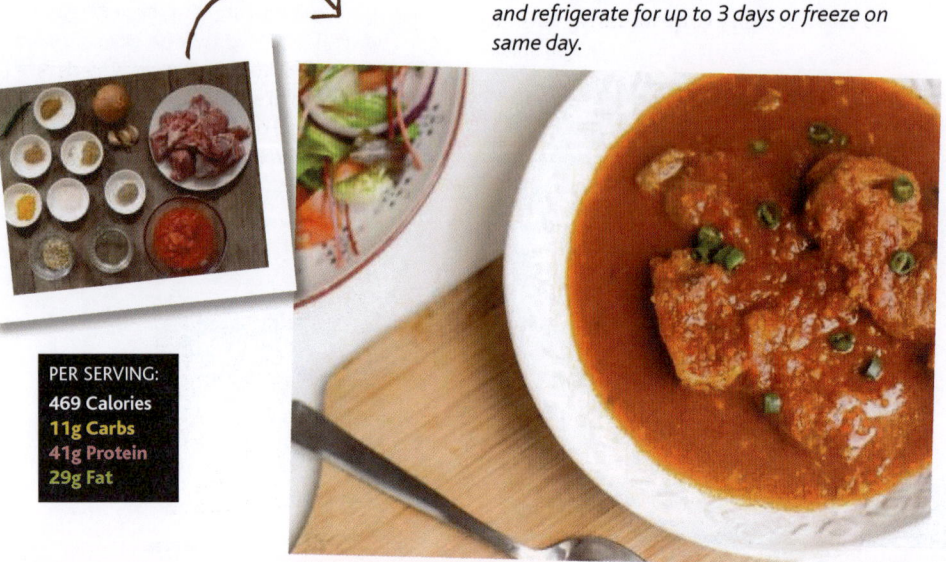

PER SERVING:
469 Calories
11g Carbs
41g Protein
29g Fat

https://thehealthandfitnesscoach.co.uk

DINNER

Cauliflower burgers

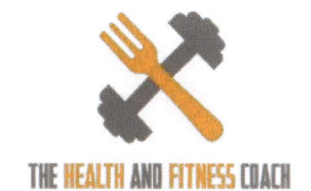

400g cauliflower, cut into florets
1 tbsp olive oil
¼ medium-sized white onion, finely chopped
2 garlic cloves, finely chopped
1 red bell-pepper, diced
1 tsp sea salt
½ tsp ground black pepper
90g ground almonds

SERVES 2

Preheat oven to 200°C/400°F. Line a baking tray with baking paper.

Place the florets onto the tray and drizzle with olive oil. Bake for 20 minutes, or until soft.

Place the onion, garlic, bell-pepper, salt, pepper and cauliflower in a food processor. Pulse gently until roughly chopped, taking care not to over process.

Transfer the mixture to a bowl and stir in the ground almonds.

Using your hands, combine the mixture into a large ball, then divide into 4 and shape into patties.

Place the patties onto the baking paper. Bake for 15-20 minutes, turning halfway through cooking time.

When the burgers are golden brown, remove them from the oven and leave to cool for 5 minutes before serving.

Store any leftovers in an airtight container and refrigerate for up to 2 days or wrap the uncooked patties individually and freeze on same day.

Serving suggestion:

Serve the burgers in a tortilla wrap, a burger bun or with a salad.

PER SERVING:
440 Calories
19g Carbs
19g Protein
32g Fat

https://thehealthandfitnesscoach.co.uk

DINNER

Chicken tagine with squash

THE HEALTH AND FITNESS COACH

2 tbsps coconut oil or ghee
2 small white onions, peeled and quartered
4 garlic cloves, minced
6cm piece of ginger, minced
½ tbsp ground coriander
1 tbsp allspice or barahat
1 tsp sea salt
1 tsp ground black pepper
1.5kg skinless bone-in chicken thighs
600ml vegetable stock (made with one organic stock cube)
1 tsp honey
500g butternut squash, cut into chunks
1 tsp cumin seeds

SERVES 6

Preheat oven to 180°C/350°F. Melt half of the oil/ghee in a large saucepan over a medium heat. Add the onions and sauté for 3-5 minutes, or until soft and translucent.

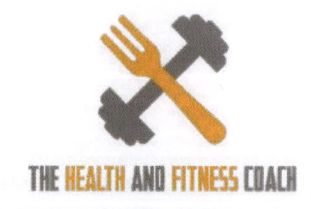

Add the garlic and ginger, stir and fry for 2 minutes, then remove from heat.

Mix the coriander, allspice, salt and pepper in a bowl. Rub the chicken with the spice mixture.

Heat the remaining oil or ghee in a medium-sized ovenproof casserole dish. Add the chicken and cook for five minutes, stirring to seal on all sides. Cook in batches if preferred.

Turn off the heat. Using tongs, arrange the chicken skin side up in the base of the dish.

Stir in the onion mixture, stock, honey, squash and cumin seeds. Bring to a gentle simmer.

Transfer to the oven and bake for 45 minutes. Serve.

Store any leftovers in an airtight container and refrigerate for up to 3 days or freeze on same day.

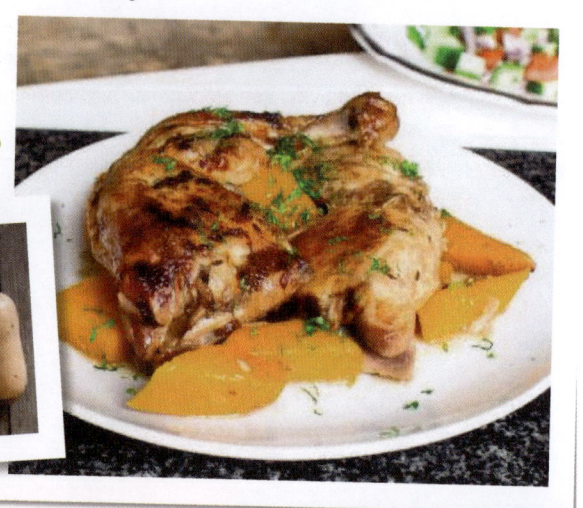

PER SERVING:
498 Calories
24g Carbs
51g Protein
22g Fat

https://thehealthandfitnesscoach.co.uk

Chickpea curry

1 tbsp olive oil or ghee
2 small white onions, finely chopped
3 garlic cloves, finely chopped
½ tbsp garam masala
1 tbsp barahat or all spice
½ tbsp ground coriander
600g tinned chopped tomatoes
600g (drained weight) tinned chickpeas, drained
1 tsp sea salt
1 tsp ground black pepper
150g fresh spinach leaves

SERVES 5

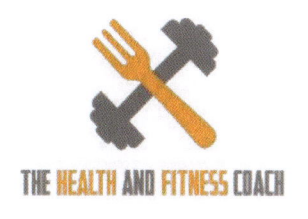

Heat the oil/ghee in a large saucepan over a medium heat. Add the onions and sauté for 3-5 minutes, stirring occasionally until translucent.

Add the garlic and fry for one minute, stirring frequently.

Add garam masala, baharat and ground coriander. Stir well and cook for one minute.

Add the chopped tomatoes, chickpeas, salt and pepper. Stir well, bring to a boil then reduce heat and simmer gently for 8 minutes.

Add the spinach and cook for two minutes, or until wilted. Serve.

Store any leftovers in an airtight container and refrigerate for up to 3 days or freeze on same day.

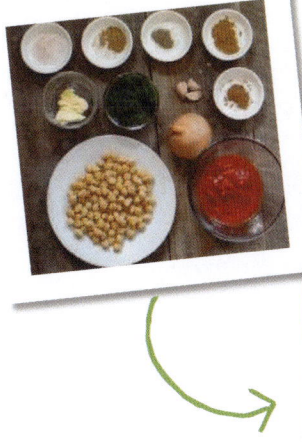

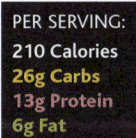

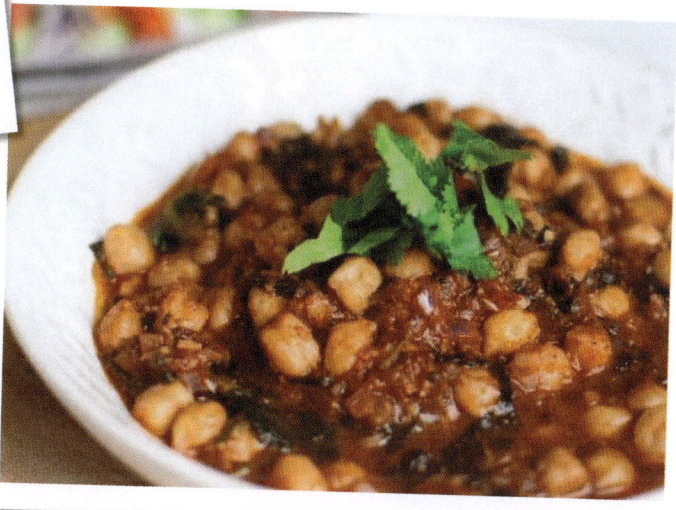

PER SERVING:
210 Calories
26g Carbs
13g Protein
6g Fat

https://thehealthandfitnesscoach.co.uk

DINNER

Veggie-rich ratatouille

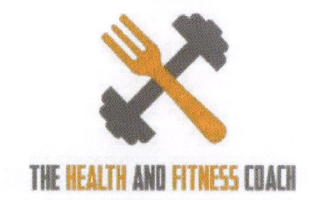

2 tbsps olive oil

for the sauce:
3 garlic cloves, minced
400g tinned chopped tomatoes
1 tsp sea salt
1 tsp ground black pepper
1 tbsp white vinegar
1 lemon, juiced
1 tbsp mixed herbs

for the vegetables:
1 aubergine, cut into 1cm thick slices
1 red bell-pepper, sliced finely
1 yellow bell-pepper, sliced finely
1 courgette, cut into 1cm thick slices
2 tomatoes, cut into 1cm thick slices

for the herb dressing:
1 garlic clove, crushed
1 tsp dried mixed herbs
1 tbsp olive oil

SERVES 8

Preheat oven to 200°C/400°F.

Heat 1 tbsp olive oil in a saucepan over a medium heat. Add the garlic and sauté for three minutes. Add the remaining sauce ingredients. Bring to a boil then reduce heat and simmer for 10 minutes. Remove the sauce from the heat and pour into a large rectangular ovenproof dish.

Arrange the vegetables around the base of the dish in alternating patterns.

Place the dressing ingredients in a jug and stir well. Gently brush the vegetables with the dressing.

Cover with foil and bake for 40 minutes. Remove the foil and bake for 15 minutes. Serve.

Store any leftovers in an airtight container and refrigerate for up to 3 days.

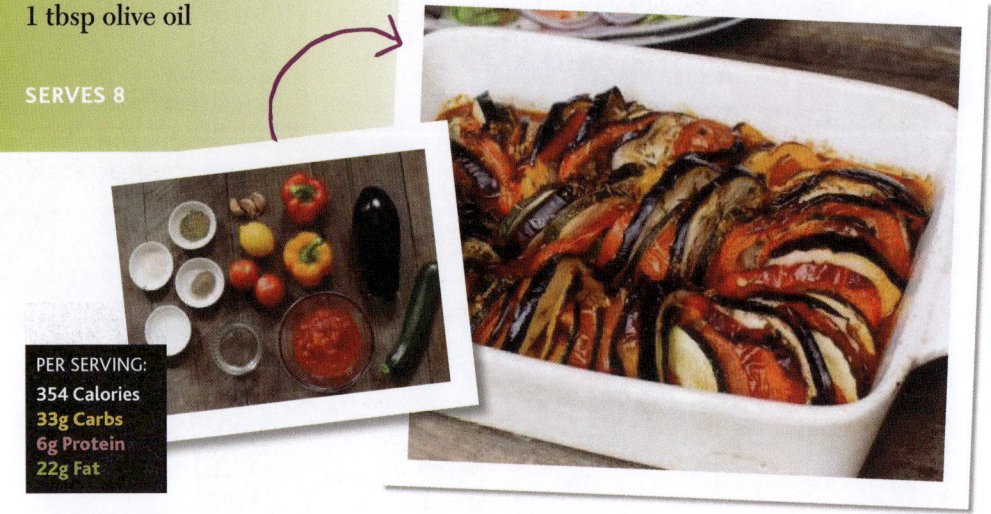

PER SERVING:
354 Calories
33g Carbs
6g Protein
22g Fat

https://thehealthandfitnesscoach.co.uk

DINNER

Baked chicken breast

300g chicken breast
½ tsp sea salt
1 tbsp dried rosemary
1 tbsp dried thyme
½ tbsp garlic powder
½ tbsp onion powder
1 tsp paprika
1 tbsp olive oil

to serve:
1 tbsp fresh parsley, finely chopped

SERVES 2

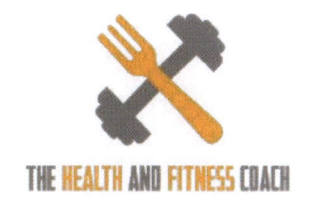

THE HEALTH AND FITNESS COACH

Preheat oven to 200°C/400°F. Line a baking tray with baking paper.

Place the chicken on a chopping board or large plate. Using a mallet or end of a wooden spoon, pound the chicken breasts ensuring they are equal thickness.

Place the dried spices in a small bowl and mix well.

Place the chicken onto the baking tray and drizzle over the olive oil. Sprinkle the mixed spices over the top and massage into the chicken.

Bake for 15-20 minutes, or until thoroughly cooked. Serve garnished with fresh parsley.

Store any leftovers in an airtight container and refrigerate for up to 3 days or freeze on same day.

Serving suggestion:

Serve the chicken on a bed of steamed rice or with a leafy salad.

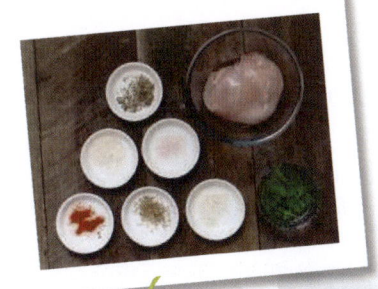

PER SERVING:
268 Calories
6g Carbs
34g Protein
12g Fat

https://thehealthandfitnesscoach.co.uk

DINNER 90

Fragrant chickpea burgers

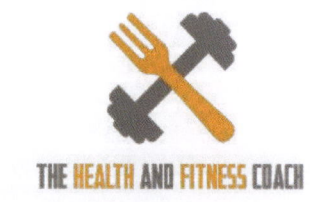

1 tbsp coconut oil
1 brioche bun per person, (optional)
for the toppings (optional):
a handful of lettuce leaves, washed
1 large ripe tomato, sliced
2 tsps (per person) mayonnaise
½ a small red onion, finely sliced
for the burgers:
250g sweet potato, peeled and diced
400g tinned chickpeas, drained
150g tinned sweetcorn, drained
1 tbsp fresh coriander
1 tsp English mustard (optional)
1 garlic clove, peeled
½ tsp paprika
½ tsp ground coriander
½ tsp ground cumin
juice of ½ a lemon
2½ tbsps plain flour (use gluten free if preferred), plus a little extra to flour surface
a pinch of sea salt and ground black pepper

Bring a small saucepan of water to the boil. Add the sweet potato and cook for 10 minutes, or until soft. Drain well and allow to cool for 15 minutes.

Place the potato and remaining burger ingredients in a food processor. Blend until well combined.

Lightly flour a surface. Shape the mixture into 5 patties on the floured surface. Dust the tops of the patties lightly with flour.

Heat half of the oil in a large frying pan over a medium/high heat. Add 2-3 patties to the pan. Reduce heat to medium and fry gently for 3-4 minutes, or until the underside is golden. Turn over and cook for 3-4 minutes. Transfer to a plate.

Repeat above step with remaining oil and patties. Serve in buns (if using) and with desired toppings.

Store any leftover burgers in an airtight container and refrigerate for up to 4 days or freeze on same day.

MAKES 5 BURGERS

PER BURGER (with bun and toppings):
376 Calories
57g Carbs
10g Protein
12g Fat

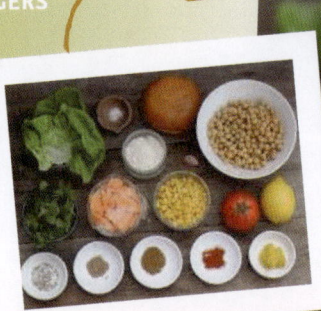

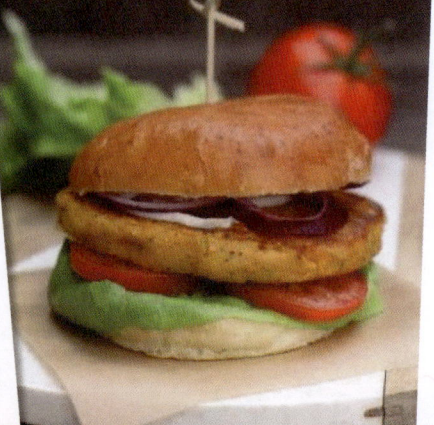

https://thehealthandfitnesscoach.co.uk

DINNER

Fragrant beef curry

2 tsps coconut oil
3 medium-sized white onions, finely chopped
6 garlic cloves, finely chopped
a thumb-sized piece of ginger, finely chopped
3-5 green chillis (depending on desired level of heat)
600g diced beef, visible fat removed
½ tsp sea salt
¼ tsp ground black pepper
1 heaped tsp madras powder
½ tsp ground turmeric
1 heaped tsp garam masala
400g tinned chopped tomatoes
2 large tomatoes, cut into segments

SERVES 4

Heat the oil in a large saucepan over a medium heat. Add the onions and fry for 4-5 minutes, stirring frequently.

Add the garlic, ginger and chillis and fry for 3 minutes, stirring frequently.

Add the beef and spices. Stir well.

Add the tinned and fresh tomatoes and stir well. Cover and cook for 40 minutes, or until the beef is tender. Stir occasionally during cooking time.

Store any leftovers in an airtight container and refrigerate for up to 4 days or freeze on same day.

Serving suggestion:

Serve on a bed of steamed rice

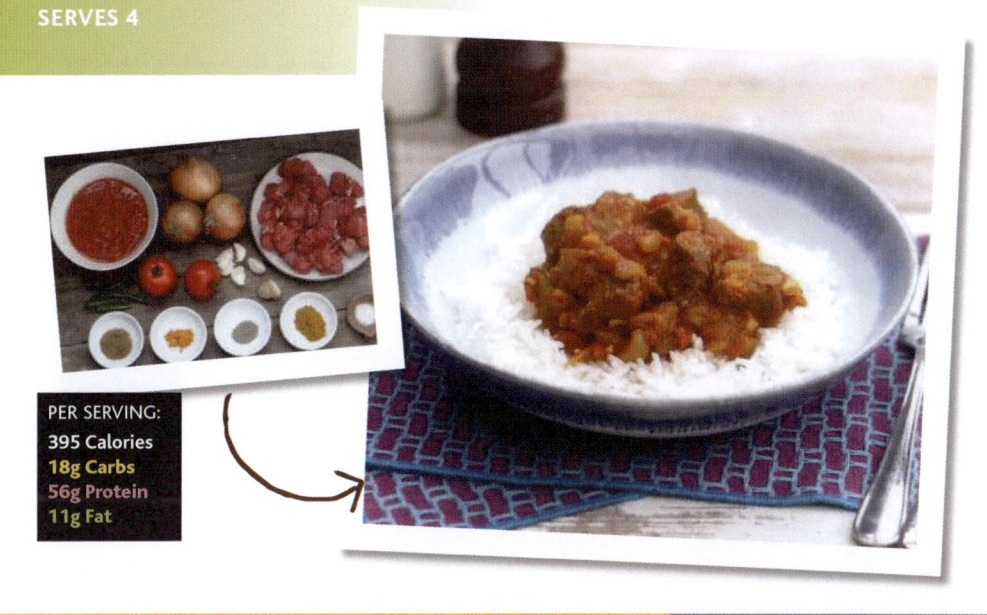

PER SERVING:
395 Calories
18g Carbs
56g Protein
11g Fat

Quick Caribbean coconut prawns

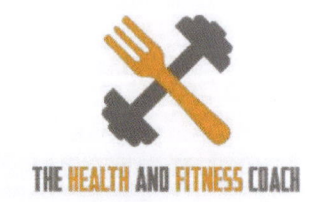

1 tsp coconut oil
1 small red onion, thinly sliced
¼-½ a small red chilli, thinly sliced
300ml coconut milk
1 tsp Jamaican jerk seasoning
300g king prawns
a small handful of fresh coriander, finely chopped

SERVES 2

Heat the coconut oil in frying pan or wok over a medium heat. Add the onion and chilli and fry for 3-4 minutes.

Stir in the coconut milk and jerk seasoning and bring to a simmer before adding the prawns. Cook for 4-5 minutes.

Serve garnished with fresh coriander.

Consume immediately.

Serving suggestion:
Serve on a bed of steamed rice

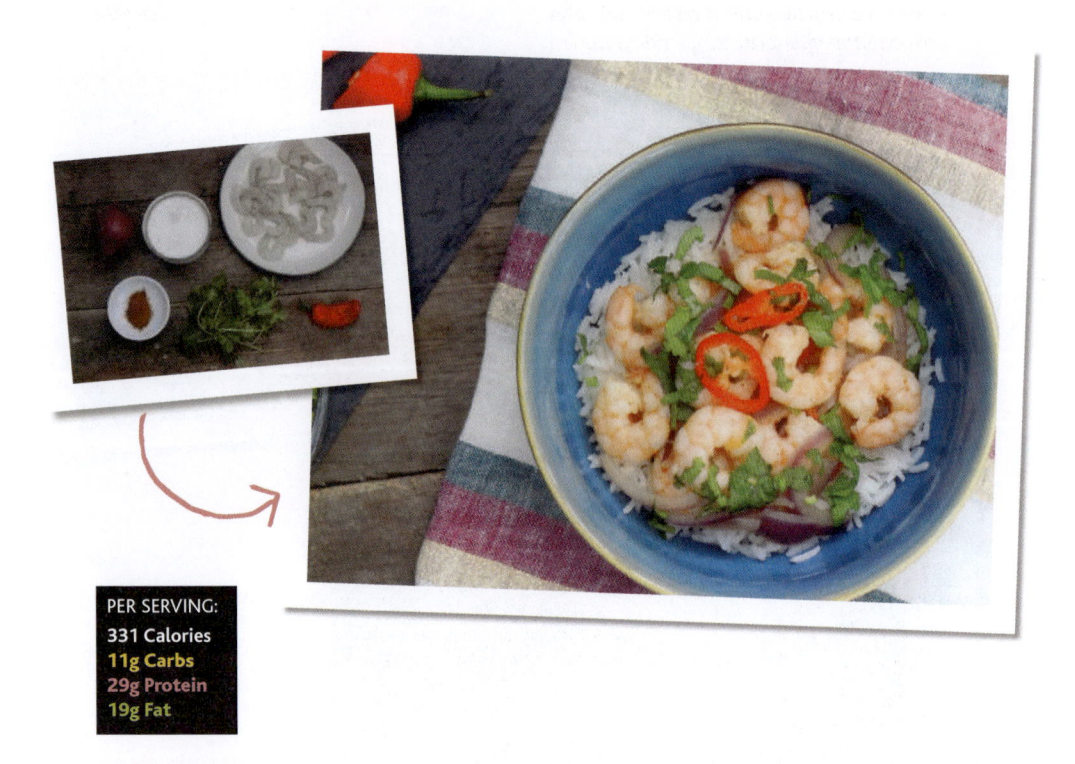

PER SERVING:
331 Calories
11g Carbs
29g Protein
19g Fat

https://thehealthandfitnesscoach.co.uk

Hearty chicken casserole

1 tbsp ghee or coconut oil
1kg skinless boneless chicken thighs
a good pinch of sea salt and ground black pepper
100g white onion, chopped
2 garlic cloves, finely chopped
2 celery sticks, sliced
300g carrots, peeled and sliced
1 large leek, sliced
500g white potatoes, peeled and diced
1 tbsp plain flour (use gluten free if preferred)
800ml hot chicken stock (made with one organic stock cube)
1 bouquet garni (available in major supermarkets)
50g uncooked quinoa (optional)

SERVES 4

Heat the ghee/oil in a large saucepan over a medium heat. Season the chicken with salt and pepper. Place in the pan and fry gently for 5 minutes on each side. Transfer to a plate and set aside.

Drain most of the excess fat from the saucepan. Add the onion, garlic, celery, carrots, leek and potatoes and fry for 5 minutes, stirring occasionally.

Stir in the flour and cook for 1 minute. Add the stock and bouquet garni.

Bring to a simmer and add the chicken. Stir gently, ensuring the chicken is covered in the liquid. Cover and simmer for 15 minutes.

Rinse the quinoa (if using) and drain well. Add it to the saucepan. Stir well and simmer for 25 minutes. Taste and add more seasoning, if required. Remove the bouquet garni and discard. Serve.

Store any leftovers in an airtight container and refrigerate for up to 4 days or freeze on same day.

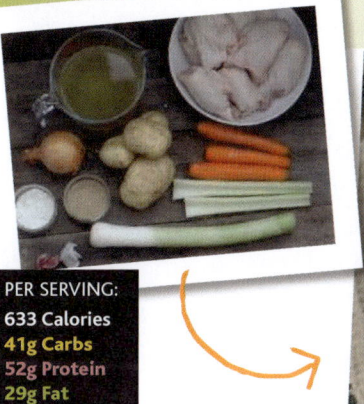

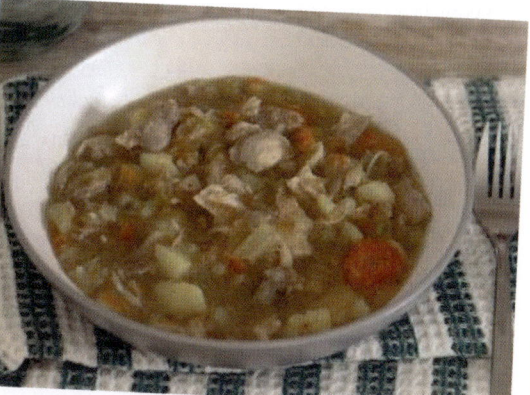

PER SERVING:
633 Calories
41g Carbs
52g Protein
29g Fat

https://thehealthandfitnesscoach.co.uk

DINNER

Quick chicken & vegetable scramble

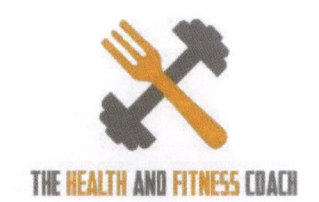

130g basmati rice
1 tsp coconut oil or ghee
1 small red onion, sliced
250g cherry tomatoes, chopped or left whole
1 garlic clove, finely chopped
a pinch of sea salt
a pinch of ground black pepper
10ml balsamic vinegar
1 tsp paprika
400g fresh chicken breast, diced
a large handful of fresh spinach leaves

SERVES 2

Bring a small saucepan of water to the boil. Add the rice, stir briefly and simmer for 20 minutes, or until the rice is cooked. Drain well.

Meanwhile, heat the oil/ghee in a frying pan over a medium/low heat. Add the onion and sauté gently for 5 minutes, stirring occasionally.

Add the tomatoes, garlic, salt, pepper, balsamic vinegar and paprika. Increase the heat to medium and cook for 4 minutes.

Transfer to a plate and set aside.

Add the chicken to the pan and cook for 5 minutes, stirring occasionally until cooked.

Add the tomato mixture back into the pan.

Add the spinach and rice and stir well. Cook for 2 minutes, stirring frequently, until the spinach has wilted. Serve.

Consume immediately.

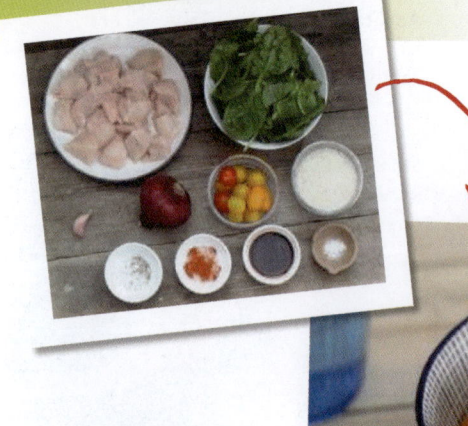

PER SERVING:
575 Calories
71g Carbs
48g Protein
11g Fat

https://thehealthandfitnesscoach.co.uk

Stuffed cabbage

300g cabbage leaves
a small handful of fresh coriander, finely chopped

for the sauce:
2 tsps olive oil
3 garlic cloves, minced
400g tinned chopped tomatoes
1 tbsp dried mixed herbs
¼ tsp sea salt
1 tbsp onion powder

for the meat filling:
300g lean beef mince
2 tsps garlic powder
1 tsp sea salt
1 tsp paprika
½ tsp cayenne pepper
1 egg, beaten

SERVES 3

Heat the oil in a saucepan over a medium flame. Add the garlic and fry gently until fragrant. Add the remaining sauce ingredients and a splash of cold water. Bring to a boil, then reduce heat and simmer for 20 minutes. Remove the sauce from the heat.

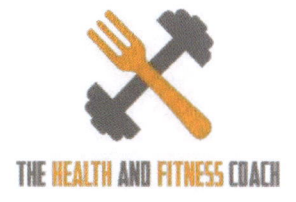

Using a stick blender, blend the sauce until smooth.

Place the meat filling ingredients in a large bowl and mix well to combine. Using a stick blender, gently blend the mixture, pulsing several times. Roll the mixture into balls, around 3 inches diameter. Set aside.

Preheat oven to 200°C/400°F.

Place the cabbage leaves in a large bowl. Cover in recently boiled water. Allow to stand for 3 minutes, to soften. Remove from the bowl using tongs and place them in a colander to cool. Place a spoonful of meat mixture onto the centre of a leaf and fold into a parcel. Repeat with the remaining meat and leaves. Place each parcel into a ceramic baking dish. Spoon the sauce over the cabbage parcels.

Cover the dish with foil and bake for 20 minutes. Remove the foil and bake for 10 minutes. Serve garnished with coriander.

Store any leftovers in an airtight container and refrigerate for up to 3 days.

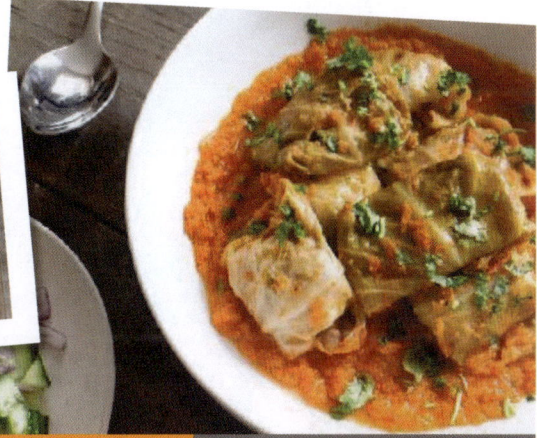

PER SERVING:
310 Calories
18g Carbs
37g Protein
10g Fat

https://thehealthandfitnesscoach.co.uk

Easy cashew chicken

25g cashews
1½ tsps coconut oil
100g white onion, roughly chopped
300g mini chicken fillets, cut into bite-sized pieces
100g green bell-pepper, roughly chopped
3 spring onions, chopped
½ tsp ground ginger
½-1 tsp ground red chilli flakes
1 tsp garlic granules
a large pinch of sea salt and ground black pepper
1 tbsp Shaosing rice wine vinegar
2 tsps soy sauce or tamari
2 tsps sesame oil
a sprinkle of sesame seeds

SERVES 2

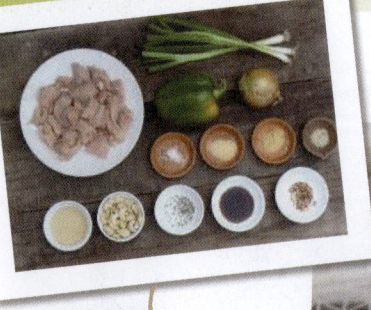

Place a frying pan over a low heat. Add the cashews and toast gently for 2-3 minutes, stirring occasionally. Remove pan from heat and allow to cool.

Place the pan back over the heat. Add half of the oil and heat until melted. Add the onion and fry gently for 4-5 minutes, stirring frequently until softened.

Add the remaining oil and increase heat to medium/high. Add the chicken and cook for 6-8 minutes, stirring frequently until cooked thoroughly.

Add the bell-pepper, spring onions, ginger, chilli flakes, garlic granules, salt and pepper. Stir well and cook for 1 minute.

Add the rice wine vinegar, soy sauce and sesame oil. Cook for 3 minutes, stirring frequently. Add the cashews, and cook for 2 minutes, stirring frequently. Serve topped with sesame seeds.

Store any leftovers in an airtight container and refrigerate for up to 3 days or freeze on same day.

PER SERVING:
432 Calories
18g Carbs
54g Protein
16g Fat

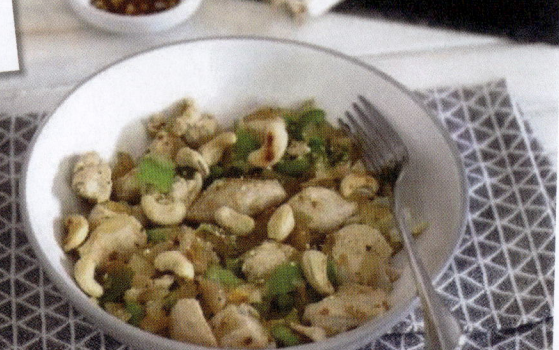

https://thehealthandfitnesscoach.co.uk

DINNER

Herby baked salmon

2 tsps butter, melted
2 garlic cloves, minced
1 tsp honey
juice of ½ lemon
½ tsp paprika
1 tbsp fresh parsley, finely chopped
⅛ tsp sea salt
⅛ tsp ground black pepper
2 x 150g fresh salmon fillets

SERVES 2

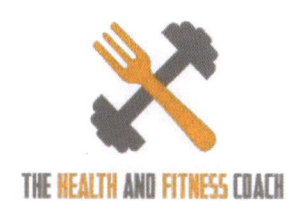

Preheat oven to 200°C/400°F.

In a bowl combine the butter, garlic, honey, lemon, paprika, parsley, salt and black pepper.

Arrange the salmon on a foil-lined baking tray. Spoon the mixture over the top of the salmon.

Bake for 15 minutes, or until the salmon is a pale pink colour throughout. Serve.

Store any leftovers in an airtight container and refrigerate for up to 2 days.

Serving suggestion:

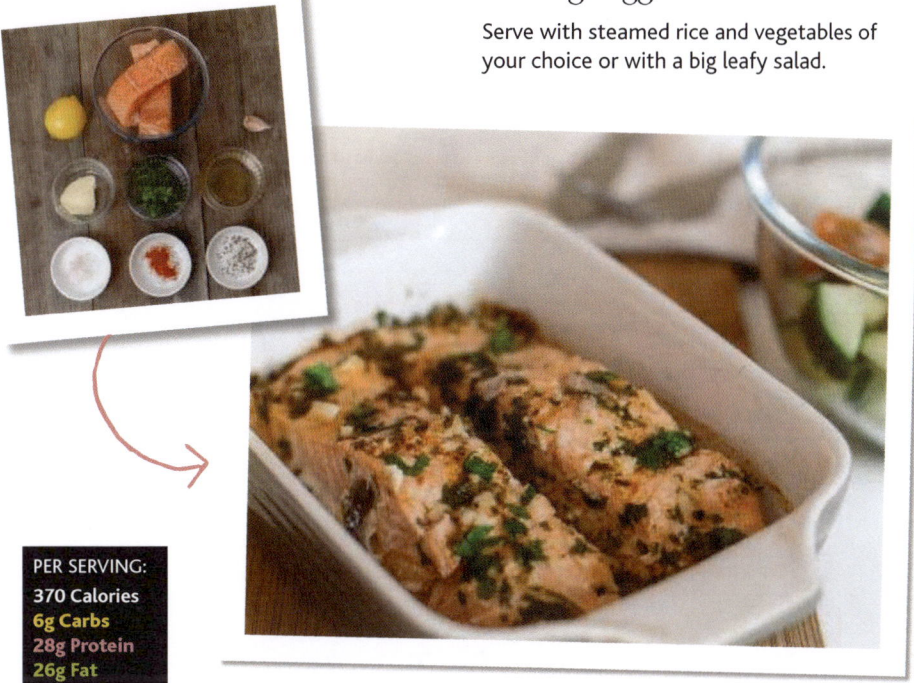

Serve with steamed rice and vegetables of your choice or with a big leafy salad.

PER SERVING:
370 Calories
6g Carbs
28g Protein
26g Fat

THE HEALTH AND FITNESS COACH

https://thehealthandfitnesscoach.co.uk

DINNER

Spiced salmon & chickpea salad

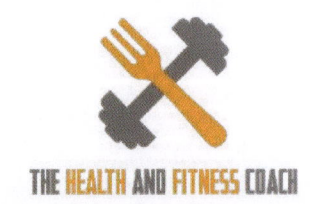

2 x 130g salmon fillets
1 tsp smoked paprika
1 tsp olive oil
½ tsp red chilli flakes
1 tsp coconut oil
1 small red onion, sliced
200g cauliflower, cut into florets
200g (drained weight) tinned chickpeas, rinsed and patted dry
2 tsps medium curry powder
100g fresh spinach leaves
8 cherry tomatoes, halved
100g cucumber, diced
2 tbsps Greek yoghurt (use dairy free if preferred)
juice of ½ a lemon
2 tsps fresh coriander, finely chopped
a pinch of sea salt and black pepper
lemon wedges, to serve

SERVES 2

Preheat oven to 200°C/400°F. Place the salmon onto a foil-lined tray. Mix the paprika, oil and chilli flakes in a bowl. Spread the mixture over the tops and sides of the salmon fillets. Bake for 20-25 minutes, or until the salmon is cooked.

Meanwhile, heat the oil in a lidded frying pan or saucepan. Add the onion and cauliflower. Stir, cover and cook for 8 minutes, stirring occasionally.

Add the chickpeas and curry powder and stir. Cook uncovered for 5 minutes, stirring occasionally. Add a small splash of water to the pan and add the spinach. Cover and cook for 2-3 minutes, or until the spinach has wilted.

Mix the tomatoes, cucumber, yoghurt, lemon juice, coriander, salt and pepper in a bowl.

Divide the chickpea mixture between two plates. Add the tomato and cucumber mixture and top with the salmon. Serve with lemon wedges.

Store any leftovers in an airtight container and refrigerate for up to 2 days.

PER SERVING:
608 Calories
36g Carbs
44g Protein
32g Fat

https://thehealthandfitnesscoach.co.uk

DINNER

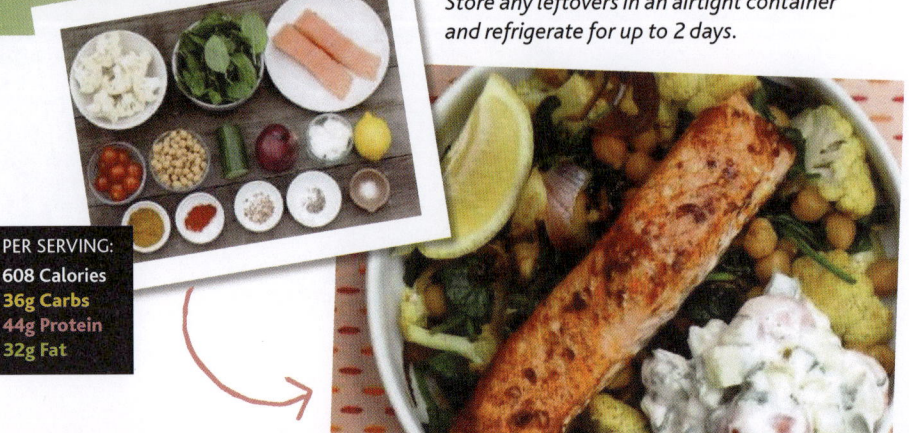

Vegetable & chickpea paella

100g short grain or arborio rice
a pinch of saffron threads
2 tsps coconut oil
1 large white onion, diced
1 red or yellow bell-pepper, sliced
250g tomato passata (or blended tinned tomatoes)
2 tbsps tomato purée
1 tsp garlic granules
½-1 tsp hot paprika
a pinch of sea salt and ground black pepper
300ml vegetable stock (made with one organic stock cube)
120g green beans, ends trimmed
200g (drained weight) tinned chickpeas, rinsed and drained well
juice of 1 lemon
a sprinkle of fresh parsley

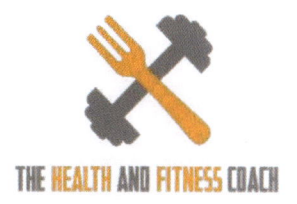

SERVES 3

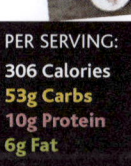

Rinse the rice in cold water. Bring a saucepan of water to the boil. Add the rice, stir briefly, and reduce heat. Simmer gently for 15-20 minutes or until the rice just begins to soften. Drain well.

Combine the saffron threads with 40ml warm water in a small bowl.

Melt the oil in a large saucepan over a medium/low heat. Add the onion and sauté for 4-5 minutes, until soft. Add the bell-pepper and cook for 5 minutes, stirring occasionally.

Add the passata, tomato purée, garlic granules, hot paprika, salt, pepper and saffron in water. Stir well and cook for 2-3 minutes. Add the green beans, chickpeas and rice and stir gently.

Add the stock and simmer gently for 15 minutes or until most of the liquid has evaporated. Add more stock during cooking time if the paella becomes too dry. Remove the saucepan from the heat, and stir in the lemon juice. Serve garnished with parsley.

Store any leftovers in an airtight container and refrigerate for up to 2 days or freeze on same day.

PER SERVING:
306 Calories
53g Carbs
10g Protein
6g Fat

https://thehealthandfitnesscoach.co.uk

DINNER

Printed in Great Britain
by Amazon